Blood Chemistry and CBC Analysis –
Clinical Laboratory Testing from a Functional Perspective

Blood Chemistry and CBC Analysis –

Clinical Laboratory Testing from a Functional Perspective

Dicken Weatherby, N.D.
Scott Ferguson, N.D.

Bear Mountain Publishing • Jacksonville, OR

Blood Chemistry and CBC Analysis- Clinical Laboratory Testing from a Functional Perspective

Bear Mountain Publishing
1-541-631-8316

ISBN 0-9761367-1-6

Warning - Disclaimer
Bear Mountain Publishing has designed this book to provide information in regard to the subject matter covered. It is sold with the understanding that the publisher and the authors are not liable for the misconception or misuse of information provided. The purpose of this book is to educate. It is not meant to be a comprehensive source for blood chemistry and CBC analysis, and is not intended as a substitute for medical diagnosis or treatment, or intended as a substitute for medical counseling. Information contained in this book should not be construed as a claim or representation that any treatment, process or interpretation mentioned constitutes a cure, palliative, or ameliorative. The interpretation is intended to supplement the practitioner's knowledge of their patient. It should be considered as adjunctive support to other diagnostic medical procedures.

Printed in the United States of America

BLOOD CHEMISTRY AND CBC ANALYSIS-
CLINICAL LABORATORY TESTING
FROM A FUNCTIONAL PERSPECTIVE

DICKEN WEATHERBY, N.D.

Dr. Dicken Weatherby is a native of England and has studied, practiced, and taught medicine in Europe and the United States. He received his Naturopathic Medical Degree from National College of Naturopathic Medicine in 1998. He is actively involved in research, writing and education, and makes his home in Southern Oregon. Dr. Weatherby is the author of *Signs and Symptoms Analysis from a Functional Perspective* and the creator of *the Blood Chemistry Software Program at* http://www.BloodChemSoftware.com

SCOTT FERGUSON, N.D.

Dr. Scott Ferguson received his Naturopathic Medical Degree in 1998 and completed his residency at National College of Naturopathic Medicine in Portland, Oregon. He is actively involved in teaching, clinical research and maintains a private practice in Portland, Orgegon. As a head consultant in the professional nutrition industry, Dr. Ferguson has worked with thousands of doctors in the field of Functional Nutrition.

Dr. Weatherby and Dr. Ferguson are the co-authors of *Blood Chemistry and CBC Analysis– Clinical Laboratory Testing from a Functional Perspective, In-Office lab testing- Functional Terrain Analysis, The Complete Practitioner's Guide to take-Home Testing,* and *The Complete Physical Exam Reporting System.*

For more information on other books by Dr. Weatherby and Dr. Ferguson please visit www.BloodChemistryAnalysis.com or e-mail Info@BloodChemistryAnalysis.com

For more information on Dr. Weatherby's Blood Chemistry Software program please visit http://www.BloodChemSoftware.com

Table of Content

SPECIAL TOPICS

APPENDIX...261

Acknowledgements

This book has incorporated information from a variety of practitioners without prejudice to degree. We have used interpretations and concepts from Western Medicine, Naturopathy, Biochemistry, and Nutrition. We would specifically like to thank the following for their contributions to our understanding of Blood Chemistry and CBC analysis.

Lynn August, MD

Dan Carter, ND

Harry Eidenier, PhD

Patricia Kane, PhD

Harold Krystal, DDS

Harold Loomis, DC

Russell Marz, ND

Joseph Montante, MD

James Said, DC, ND

Steven Sandberg-Lewis, ND

Alexander Schauss, Ph.D.

Guy Schenker, DC

John Sherman, ND

Dickson Thom, DDS, ND

Introduction

Most of us are using the conventional laboratory reference ranges for our blood chemistry and CBC interpretation. For many practitioners blood chemistry and CBC analysis is a matter of comparing a test result with the conventional laboratory reference range, seeing whether or not the patient's results are normal or abnormal and attempting to fit them into a particular disease pattern or pathology. Unfortunately these conventional laboratory ranges are designed to identify and diagnose disease states and pathology. People who fall within the reference range are assumed to have no clinical signs and symptoms of any disease, and are considered "normal".

In the field of alternative and preventative medicine we know that most of our patients are by no means "normal", so why do we use an interpretive method that is based on that assumption? It is our hope that this book will present another method of analysis, one that looks at blood chemistries from a functional or prognostic perspective and can therefore give us data on how the physiology of body is functioning. By looking for optimum function we increase our ability to detect the dysfunctions that plague our patients long before disease manifests. Our conventional lab testing becomes more comprehensive by being prognostic and preventative, as well as pathology oriented.

Functional versus pathological

Medicine and health care are undergoing a paradigm shift. We are seeing more and more demand from our patients to look at their complex cases from a holistic rather than a mechanistic or reductionistic perspective. In order to do this we need to have diagnostic methods that focus on physiological function as a marker of health, rather than merely the presence of pathology or tissue change as a marker of disease. The following lists the differences between a reductionistic, pathological view of the body, and the view of the body as functioning physiology.

PATHOLOGICAL VIEW

1. The body is viewed as a "machine" composed of separate systems reduced into its constituent parts.
2. Emphasis is placed on the identification of disease or pathological tissue change.
3. Diagnosis is extremely specialized.
4. Treatment is based on reducing symptoms.
5. Major focus is spent on how the patient is doing based on charts, statistics, and test results etc. that are measured against a statistical "normal population".

FUNCTIONAL VIEW

1. The body is viewed as a dynamic and complex interconnected system of mind, body, and emotions.
2. Emphasis is placed on identification of areas of imbalance or dysfunction in normal physiology.
3. Diagnosis integrates data from many different systems and methods.
4. Treatment addresses the underlying causes of dysfunction.
5. Major focus is spent on both subjective and objective information gathering based on a concept of optimal physiological function.

PATHOLOGICAL VIEW	**FUNCTIONAL VIEW**
6. Relies on late stage development of disease as a marker.	6. Allows for an early prediction of dysfunction.
7. Health is measured as an absence of disease. As long as you do not have a disease, you are considered healthy.	7. Health is measured along a wellness continuum, which is a spectrum moving from health to disease. Intervention can be made at every stage of the spectrum to restore and/or improve health and wellness.

The main focus of this book is to look at blood chemistry and CBC testing from this functional perspective. We will present different ranges, which we call optimal ranges, for each test on a regular blood chemistry and CBC or hematology screen. In addition to the US units of measurement we have included the Standard International units used by physicians in the rest of the world.

Alternative blood chemistry and CBC analysis has been around for many years with many researchers and clinicians contributing their particular talents to this growing field. We have been using this particular method of analysis for the last 6 years, and over that time we have refined our diagnostic criteria into the system that it is today.

Conventional Laboratory Reference Ranges vs., Optimal Ranges

Conventional laboratory reference ranges are designed to identify and diagnose disease states and pathology. People who fall within the reference range are assumed to have no clinical signs and symptoms of any disease, and are considered "normal". The reference range used by conventional laboratories is based on a Gaussian or bell curve distribution of test results with an established mean value. The standard in laboratory medicine is to use 2 standard deviations above and below the mean to represent normal. This places 95% of people within the "clinically" normal reference range.

Unfortunately, this method of assessment does not allow for the large numbers of people who are told that they are "clinically" normal yet suffer from a wide range of signs and symptoms more suggestive of a subclinical or functional problem. The conventional reference ranges, because they are based on the Gaussian distribution, get wider and wider as the population gets sicker and sicker. Remember 95% of the population falls within the normal reference range. As the population becomes sicker the number of people who are declared "clinically normal" gets larger, making the definition of abnormal or disease states relative.

It is our experience that most people who seek medical care do not have a clinically identifiable disease. As a result they are told by their doctor that they have an "unremarkable" or "normal" laboratory test, i.e. they are "clinically" normal. They may be normal compared to the rest of the sick population, but they are a long way from being in a state of optimal health.

Many of the optimal ranges in this book used to be the "normal" ranges 10 or 15 years ago. Also, many of these optimal ranges and patterns were inadvertently discovered by doctors seeking serum cancer markers. The optimal ranges are tighter than the conventional laboratory reference ranges, thereby increasing the sensitivity while reducing specificity. We increase our ability to detect patients with changes in physiological function and thus use laboratory testing in a more preventative way. We can identify the factors that obstruct the patient from achieving optimal physiological, biochemical, and metabolic functioning in their body. For example, if a patient's blood glucose is 105 mg/dL or 5.82 mmol/L., this falls within the normal laboratory reference range. In the conventional system the patient would be told that the lab test is normal and that he/she does not have diabetes. This is true, the patient may not have diabetes now, but as functionally-oriented practitioners we are more concerned with preventing disease from occurring. By using an optimal range for blood glucose, a serum glucose of 105 mg/dL or 5.82 mmol/L alerts us to the possibility that this patient's ability to regulate blood glucose is becoming compromised. Combining this with a thorough history, a diet and symptom analysis, functional physical exam, and looking at other values on their chemistry screen we can more accurately determine whether or not the patient is having problems with blood sugar dysregulation. We have the opportunity to deal with the dysfunction long before it manifests in diabetes.

Patterns/trends

We have added sections throughout the book on the key patterns and trends that exist between different laboratory tests. The body's blood chemistry is a profound network of checks and balances, biochemical regulation of function, and important compensatory mechanisms at work. To analyze only an isolated value or limited set of values is therefore incomplete. Often what we see in our patients is the result of something else that's out of balance, rather than the apparent problem itself. The detective work is simplified by understanding the root cause of many chemistry shifts and observing key trends and patterns suggestive of metabolic dysfunction long before there is overt pathology.

We must therefore learn to recognize and treat the underlying cause of these imbalances and not just the compensatory reactions occurring in response. Treatment of a metabolic or nutritional dysfunction at the root level will produce a more efficient and longer lasting result than just treating one symptom or effect of the imbalance.

In addition, independent values can be used to track particular trends (i.e. lipid levels); however, we propose looking at all values in the context of many other related values or clusters (i.e. lipid levels and serum glucose for Metabolic Syndrome) in order to establish causative patterns which can direct the clinician to key diagnostic and therapeutic resources.

Where blood chemistries fit in the scope of practice

Many practitioners base their treatment decisions and follow-up care primarily on symptoms and patient history alone, because many lab tests, when analyzed using the conventional laboratory reference range, are "normal" and are often too expensive to repeat frequently. This is unfortunate, because many symptoms emerge later into a process of dysfunction or pathology and often disappear long before a dysfunction is fully addressed. This leaves a large prognostic "gray zone" both before and after a symptom is present.

It is essential in a practice of patient-centered preventative medicine to have the tools to assess where a patient lies upon this spectrum. Blood chemistry and CBC analysis from an optimal and functional perspective is one of the tools that allows the practitioner to assess that prognostic "gray zone". We also recommend using symptom questionnaires, a thorough functional physical examination, and appropriate in-office lab tests along with regular blood chemistry analysis to get a thorough picture of what is going on.

Incorporating symptom questionnaires into the analysis can be very useful. We cannot over-emphasize the importance of a good, thorough history when interpreting baseline or serial laboratory values. Diet, lifestyle, and medication history is critical for the proper interpretation of a routine blood analysis, as many of these factors play an important role in establishing the etiology of a dysfunction.

We recommend running a comprehensive blood chemistry and CBC every 6 months for active patients and every year for those patients on a maintenance program. They should be run more frequently when dealing with an acute case. In between these visits we encourage the use of simple and inexpensive in-office laboratory tests that can be run economically to help track a patient's progress. Recommendations for these tests are made throughout the book. Please see our book entitled "*In-Office Lab Testing-Functional Terrain Analysis*" for a more comprehensive and detailed explanation of these in-office tests.

Most tests do not give immediate feedback and therefore take valuable time between data gathering and action or treatment. In our office we use a biofeedback technique called Neuro-Lingual Testing in conjunction with hands-on reflex testing to quickly and accurately gather data from the patient. We find that this system of analysis, when combined with blood chemistry and CBC analysis and appropriate in-office testing, allows us to accurately assess the individual needs of the patient.

For more information on health questionnaires, in-office lab testing, Neuro-Lingual Testing, and the hands-on reflex testing please see the resources pages at the back of this book or call 541-631-8316

Procedure and Integration into Practice

This method of blood chemistry analysis will help you elucidate multiple nutritional and metabolic deficiencies as well as identify potential organ dysfunction. We therefore advocate doing a full comprehensive metabolic panel in addition to a complete blood count and differential on all patients for a proper analysis. Please note that many laboratories are variable in their nomenclature, methodologies, and order of reporting values. Standard international units are included throughout our material for your conversion if needed.

We recommend a full chemistry panel and CBC on every patient to:

      1. Establish working baseline if they have not had recent testing.

2. To assess their current health status and identify patterns or trends from previous testing.

3. To use as a prognostic indicator for potential nutritional and/or metabolic imbalances and to establish a preventative health plan.

We recommend that you run a full chemistry panel and CBC every six months for active patients and every year for patients on a maintenance program.

Explanation of Icons

	This icon represents a clinical implication or topic that is more **Naturopathic** in its approach.
	This icon is used to represent less common **Naturopathic** implications or to draw your attention to special areas in the body of the text.
	This icon represents a clinical implication or topic that is a more **allopathic** in its approach.
	This icon alerts the reader to either a special topic box or **drugs/medications** that are associated with increased or decreased values of a lab component.
	This icon alerts the reader to clinical implications that should be **referred** to a physician qualified to dealing with that situation.
	This icon alerts the reader to conditions that may be a **medical emergency**.
	This icon alerts the reader to a **rare** condition that should be considered but not with a high priority.

BLOOD CHEMISTRY SCREEN

Blood/Serum Glucose

Background

The level of glucose in the blood is primarily dependent on the liver, which exerts a considerable influence through the breakdown of glycogen, and via the adrenal glands, which produce hormones that promote the gluconeogenesis of fats and proteins. Glucose is also directly formed in the body from carbohydrate digestion and from the conversion in the liver of other sugars, such as fructose, into glucose.

Discussion

 The regulatory mechanisms that help control blood glucose levels are complex, involving an intricate system of inter-connecting hormones.

- **Insulin**, secreted from the beta islet cells in the pancreas, transports glucose into the cells by increasing the permeability of glucose through the cellular membrane. In addition, insulin stimulates fat, protein and glycogen synthesis. The sum of insulin activity in the body is to decrease blood glucose levels.

- **Glucagon**, on the other hand, acts on the liver to cause glycogen breakdown and thus serves to increase blood glucose levels.

- Blood glucose levels are also influenced by a number of different hormones, including epinephrine, cortisol, thyroxine, which tends to act on the liver to elevate blood glucose.

- The test for blood sugar is used to detect disorders of metabolism that may be the result of one of several causes:

    1. Inability of the beta islet cells of the pancreas to produce insulin.

    2. Reduced number of insulin receptors on target cells (increased peripheral resistance)

    3. Inability of the intestines to absorb glucose

    4. Inability of the liver to accumulate and break down glycogen

    5. The presence of increasing amounts of hormones that directly influence the liver e.g. ACTH, epinephrine, cortisol

Ranges:

	Standard U.S. Units	Standard International Units
Conventional Laboratory Range	65 – 115 mg/dl	3.61 – 6.38 mmol/L
Optimal Range	80 – 100 mg/dL	4.44 – 5.55 mmol/L
Alarm Ranges	< 50 or > 250 mg/dl	< 2.78 or > 13.88 mmol/L

When would you run this test?

1. Screening for potential dysglycemia and blood sugar dysregulation in conjunction with a full chem. screen and Glucose Tolerance Test with or without insulin

2. Diabetes management- this test is a vital component of any diabetes management program.

NOTE: Single fasting blood glucose levels are not a good screening tool for diabetes. Follow-up abnormal readings with a glucose tolerance test with or without insulin to confirm a diagnosis.

Clinical implications

HIGH

Clinical Implication	Additional information
Insulin resistance (Early stage) and glucose intolerance	Research has shown that individuals progress through several stages of insulin resistance and glucose intolerance before becoming a classic type II diabetic. The stages include: Normal glucose tolerance → hypoglycemia (often due to hyperinsulinemia) → insulin insensitivity/resistance → eventually overt type II diabetes. An increased blood glucose level is a sign that this individual is possibly in the insulin resistant phase, also known as a pre-diabetic state.
Early stage of Hyperglycemia/Diabetes	A diagnosis of diabetes mellitus requires a fasting plasma glucose level of > 140mg/dl (7.77 mmol/L) on more than one occasion. Elevated blood glucose above the optimal range (> 100 or 5.55 mmol/L) is a sign that this person may be moving down that road. If blood glucose is increased, follow-up with Hemoglobin A1C or glycated hemoglobin.

	Pattern: If serum glucose (> 100 or 5.55 mmol/L) and Hemoglobin A1C (> 5.7% or 0.057) are both elevated, diabetes is **probable**. Serum triglycerides are often higher than the total cholesterol level in diabetes. Urinary glucose may be increased (>100 or 5.55 mmol/L), HDL levels decreased (< 55 or < 1.42 mmol/L), BUN (> 16 or 5.71 mmol/L) and creatinine (>1.1 or >97.2 μmol/dL) frequently increased with the renal damage associated with diabetes. Follow-up with appropriate testing to confirm the diagnosis, e.g. oral glucose tolerance testing. Most people who are becoming insulin resistant and whose fasting blood glucose levels are starting to increase have no or very few symptoms. Some of the classic signs and symptoms of hyperglycemia include: 1. Poor wound healing 2. Frequent thirst 3. Frequent urination 4. Family history of diabetes 5. Obesity 6. Excessive hunger 7. Visual changes
Metabolic Syndrome/ hyperinsulinemia 	Metabolic Syndrome or hyperinsulinemia is a cluster of related symptoms: Increased triglycerides (>110 or >1.24 mmol/L), total cholesterol (>220 or 5.69 mmol/L), decreased HDL cholesterol (< 55 or < 1.42 mmol/L), obesity, increased blood insulin levels, increased glucose (> 100 or 5.55 mmol/L) and increased blood pressure. The hallmark of this syndrome is the insulin resistance that leads to high glucose levels and an imbalance in blood fats. The overall effect is an increased risk for cardiovascular disease and diabetes. **Please see the special topic on Metabolic Syndrome on page 9 for more information.**
Thiamine (Vitamin B1) need 	An increased glucose (> 100 or 5.55 mmol/L) is associated with a thiamine need. Thiamine transports glucose across the blood brain barrier and is an essential component in the enzymatic conversion of pyruvate into acetyl CoA that allows pyruvate to enter the Kreb's cycle. **Please see the special topic on thiamine deficiency on page 82 for more details.**

	Pattern:
	
	  If glucose is only moderately increased (> 100 or 5.55 mmol/L) and the hemoglobin A1C is normal, thiamine need is **possible**.
	
	  If CO_2 is decreased (<25) and the anion gap is increased (>12) along with moderately high serum glucose (>100 or 5.55 mmol/L), thiamine need is **probable**. Due to thiamine's role in glycolysis, LDH levels may be decreased (<140).

Anterior Pituitary resistance to cortisol 	During the decompensated/maladapted phase of the chronic stress response, the hypothalamus and pituitary become less and less sensitive to cortisol, causing increased cortisol resistance. The net result is an increase in cortisol levels in the body because the negative feedback loop that shuts cortisol production down is not activated. Increased levels of circulating cortisol will cause increased blood glucose levels through increased gluconeogenesis. Excess cortisol will also reduce the utilization and uptake of glucose by the cell.
Acute Stress 	Increasing levels of stress cause the body to move into the chronic stress response. This is marked by an increased Cortisol to DHEA ratio, which causes an increase in gluconeogenic activity and a concomitant rise in blood glucose levels. Excess cortisol will also reduce the utilization and uptake of glucose by the cell.
Fatty liver (early development) and Liver congestion 	High blood glucose (>100 or 5.55 mmol/L) levels have been associated with increased levels of blood fats, e.g. high total cholesterol (>220 or 5.69 mmol/L), LDL (>120 or 3.1 mmol/L) and triglycerides (>110 or >1.24 mmol/L), low HDL (< 55 or < 1.42 mmol/L). In individuals with liver congestion, this may lead to the deposition of fat in the liver and the development of fatty liver. Fatty liver is caused by obesity, excessive alcohol consumption, prescription drugs (e.g. steroids), iron overload, solvent exposure, and rapid weight loss. Fatty changes to the liver tissue can impair the liver's detoxification ability. The degree of fatty liver changes is directly related to the amount of obesity. **Pattern:** If total cholesterol (>220 or 5.69 mmol/L), LDL (>120 or 3.1 mmol/L), glucose (> 100 or 5.55 mmol/L) and triglyceride levels (>110 or >1.24 mmol/L) are increased,

	and HDL levels (< 55 or < 1.42 mmol/L) are decreased, then the early development of fatty liver is **possible**.
	🫀 Liver congestion, due to the fatty liver, should be considered if total cholesterol is above 220 or 5.69 mmol/L, triglycerides are increased (>110 or >1.24 mmol/L), and the SGPT/ALT is below 10.
	Fatty liver and liver congestion increases the risk of insulin resistance, hypertension, Metabolic Syndrome, and type II diabetes.
Obesity	Obesity is strongly associated with type II diabetes.
Drug causes of ⬆	❋ Corticosteroids ❋ Phenytoin ❋ Estrogen ❋ Thiazides
Other conditions associated with increased Glucose levels include	❋ Acute pancreatitis ❋ Hyperthyroidism ❋ Cushing's disease (increased levels of Glucocorticoids will elevate blood glucose) ❋ Pituitary adenoma (can lead to increased growth hormone levels, which will ⬆ blood glucose) ❋ Adenoma of pancreas, myocardial infarction ❋ Acute physical stress situations ❋ Brain damage ❋ Severe liver disease ❋ Severe renal disease ❋ Pregnancy

LOW

Clinical Implication	Additional information
Hypoglycemia-reactive	A decreased fasting blood glucose (<80 or 4.44 mmol/L) along with a decreased LDH (<140) is a common finding in reactive hypoglycemia. Hemoglobin A1C levels may also be decreased (<4.1% or 0.041). LDH is an important enzyme for pyruvate metabolism in glycolysis and is associated with pancreatic function and glucose metabolism. Suspect hypoglycemia if there are strong subjective indicators: 1. Strong craving for sweets (especially true for reactive hypoglycemia) 2. Awaken a few hours after sleeping, hard to get back to sleep

	3. Crave coffee or sweets in the afternoon
	4. Sleepy in the afternoon
	5. Fatigue relieved by eating
	6. Headache if meals are skipped or delayed
	7. Irritable before meals
	8. Shaky if meals are delayed
	Low blood pressure is a common finding with hypoglycemia and may be caused by adrenal insufficiency. A 5-6 hour oral glucose tolerance test with or without insulin levels may be necessary to determine if the patient is suffering from reactive hypoglycemia.
	If a glucose tolerance test is completed and there is evidence of a "flat curve", a heavy metal body burden is possible. Often with a heavy metal body burden or exposure to toxins, LDH-5 isoenzyme fraction will be decreased below 6%.
Hypoglycemia- liver glycogen problem	A decreased ability of the liver to store and/or produce glycogen can be a major cause of fasting low blood sugar and hypoglycemia, especially if SGPT/ALT is high (>30).
	According to Dick Thom, N.D. "The patient with this type of hypoglycemia wakes up groggy, they need 3 cups of coffee to get started and can then go for hours without eating. They seem to get by with coffee and an occasional donut for lunch. In the evening they eat a huge meal and collapse asleep. They feel bad on the weekends and cannot tolerate vacation because they feel lousy. They have to have some type of stress in their lives in order to keep going because they need the cortisol release to stimulate the liver to release glycogen. Without it they cannot keep up. "
Hyperinsulinism	A diet high in refined carbohydrates can lead to excessive secretion of insulin. High levels of circulating insulin can depress blood glucose levels to the point of hypoglycemia. An increased simple sugar intake leads first to hypoglycemia and later to diabetes. Studies have demonstrated that the persistent consumption of refined sugars and the resulting increase in blood insulin levels eventually lead to the development of type II diabetes.
Adrenal hypofunction	Adrenal fatigue leads to a decreased output of cortisol, a hormone that functions to increase blood sugar when blood sugar levels are low.

Drug causes of ↓	Alcohol	
	Insulin	
	Propranolol	
	Oral hypoglycemic drugs: sulfonylureas, tolbutamide, metformin	
Other conditions associated with decreased Glucose levels include	Pancreatic tumors	Hypofunction of anterior pituitary
	Extra-pancreatic tumors	Liver damage
	Addison's disease	Enzyme deficiency diseases (galactosemia, maple syrup disease)
	Hypothyroidism	

Interfering Factors:

Falsely increased levels	Falsely decreased levels
• Blood with a low hematocrit (<35%) may have a higher result (by about 10-15%) • Pregnancy (usually a slight elevation is seen)	• Blood with a high hematocrit (>55%) may have a lower result • Capillary measurements from cyanotic areas

Related Tests:

Serum triglycerides, total cholesterol, hemoglobin A1C, blood insulin, urine glucose, glucose tolerance test with or without insulin, HDL, LDL and VLDL cholesterol

What is Metabolic Syndrome?

Syndrome "X" was a term that was first used by Gerald Reaven, M.D., a researcher at Stanford University, to describe a cluster of interrelated symptoms that seemed to appear in individuals and increase their risk of cardiovascular disease. It has subsequently become known as Metabolic Syndrome. The syndrome is characterized by the following: high triglycerides, high cholesterol, decreased HDL cholesterol, increased serum insulin, high blood pressure, and glucose intolerance. The underlying factor in Metabolic Syndrome is elevated insulin levels and insulin resistance. All other factors are secondary to this.

Insulin resistance occurs when insulin released from the pancreas is no longer able to "unlock" the door that allows the glucose to move into the cell. It is caused by the over-consumption of refined carbohydrates, sugars and trans fatty acids in the form of hydrogenated oil. Under normal circumstances the body is able to break down carbohydrates into glucose, release adequate amounts of insulin and up-take the glucose into the cell where it is converted into ATP. Metabolic Syndrome starts when the body can no longer handle the over-consumption of refined carbohydrates and sugars day in and day out that causes the insulin levels in the blood to remain high and the cells to become less and less responsive and more and more resistant to insulin's effect. The net effect is that glucose levels remain high, which increases the likelihood of protein glycosylation and oxidative stress from free radical production, both of which have been linked with aging and the development of chronic degenerative diseases. Excessive insulin or hyperinsulinemia is a risk factor for the development of atherosclerosis, type II diabetes, obesity, some forms of dementia, and other diseases.

Insulin resistance sets the stage for the development of more serious metabolic issues. Blood triglycerides cholesterol and glucose levels begin to rise, the HDL levels begin to drop and the patient begins to put on weight and their blood pressure begins to rise.

Metabolic Syndrome, along with hypoglycemia, increased insulin secretion, and type II diabetes are all progressions of the same problem. The over-consumption of refined carbohydrates, sugars, and hydrogenated oils causes insulin resistance.

Insulin resistance takes many years to become severe. As alternative physicians we play an essential role in preventing this cascade from occurring by paying attention to some of the early warning signs: increasing blood glucose, cholesterol and triglyceride levels, decreasing HDL levels and by monitoring blood pressure. It is essential to reduce your patient's intake of refined carbohydrates, sugars, trans fatty acids and other harmful compounds. By doing this with your patients in their 30s or 40s, you can reverse insulin resistance and prevent diabetes and coronary heart disease.

Hemoglobin A1C or Glycosylated Hemoglobin

Background

During the normal lifespan of a red blood cell, which is about 120 days, glucose combines with the hemoglobin to produce a substance called glycohemoglobin. The amount of glycohemoglobin formed is in direct proportion to the amount of glucose present in the blood stream during the 120-day red blood cell lifespan. In the presence of high blood glucose levels (hyperglycemia) the amount of hemoglobin that is glycosylated to form glycohemoglobin increases. The process of glycosylation is irreversible. In short, the longer blood glucose levels remain high and the greater the amount of glucose in the blood, the more the glucose will attach to the red blood cells.

Discussion

The hemoglobin A1C test reflects the amount of non-enzymatic glycosylation that occurs on a minor sub-type of hemoglobin called A1C. It shows the average levels of blood glucose in a 2-3 month period before the test.

- It is used primarily to monitor long-term blood glucose control and to help determine therapeutic options for treatment and management. Studies have shown that the closer to normal the hemoglobin A1C levels are kept, the less likely those patients are to develop the long-term complications of diabetes.

- This test is a poor screening test for diabetes. An oral glucose tolerance test with or without insulin is the preferred screening test for diabetes.

Note:

Different labs may use different tests to determine glycosylated hemoglobin. The most common and most specific test measures hemoglobin A1C levels. Other tests may have different values. Check with your lab to determine what type of test they are doing for glycosylated hemoglobin and what their values are.

Ranges: The results are expressed as a percentage of total hemoglobin.

	Standard U.S. Units	Standard International Units
Conventional Laboratory Range	<7%	0.07
Optimal Range	4.1 – 5.7%	0.041 – 0.057

When would you run this test?

1. To follow long-term blood glucose control. It can be used to check up on diabetic patients to see whether or not they are managing their blood glucose levels between office visits. You may have patients with diabetes who change their dietary habits etc. before their scheduled appointments, so that their blood glucose control appears better than it actually is.

2. To check on the pre-diabetic patient to ensure that they are keeping their glucose levels within the optimal range.

3. To screen for hypoglycemia.

4. To determine the therapeutic choices and directions for diabetes management.

5. To follow up on diabetic patients whose renal threshold for glucose is abnormal.

6. To follow insulin dependent diabetics whose blood glucose levels fluctuate from day to day.

Clinical implications

HIGH

Clinical Implication	Additional information	
Diabetes mellitus	This test is a measurement of long-term blood glucose control and management. Values will be increased in patients with poorly controlled diabetes. It is important to remember that a patient who has recently made the changes to control their short-term blood glucose levels may still show elevated levels of glycosylated hemoglobin.	
Insulin resistance (early stage) and glucose intolerance	An increased hemoglobin A1C above the optimal range (>5.7% or >0.057) is a sign that this individual is not controlling their long term glucose levels very well. They are possibly in the insulin resistant phase, also known as a pre-diabetic state.	
	Research has shown that individuals progress through several stages of insulin resistance and glucose intolerance before becoming a classic type II diabetic. The stages include:	
	Normal glucose tolerance → hypoglycemia (often due to hyperinsulinemia) → insulin insensitivity/resistance → eventually overt type II diabetes.	
Other conditions associated with ↑ Hemoglobin A1C	✳ Splenectomy	✳ Alcohol
	✳ Iron deficiency anemia	✳ Lead toxicity

LOW

Clinical Implication	Additional information	
Hypoglycemia	A low hemoglobin A1C (<4.1% or 0.041) may be caused by an inability to maintain adequate long-term levels of glucose. A decreased fasting blood glucose (<80 or 4.44 mmol/L) along with a decreased LDH (<140) is a common finding in reactive hypoglycemia. LDH is an important enzyme for pyruvate metabolism in glycolysis and is associated with pancreatic function and glucose metabolism.	
	Suspect hypoglycemia if there are strong subjective indicators:	
	1. Strong craving for sweets (especially true for reactive hypoglycemia) 2. Awaken a few hours after sleeping, hard to get back to sleep 3. Crave coffee or sweets in the afternoon 4. Sleepy in the afternoon 5. Fatigue relieved by eating 6. Headache if meals are skipped or delayed 7. Irritable before meals & shaky if meals are delayed	
	Low blood pressure is a common finding with hypoglycemia and may be caused by adrenal insufficiency. A 5-6 hour oral glucose tolerance test with or without insulin levels may be necessary to check for reactive hypoglycemia.	
Other conditions associated with decreased Hemoglobin A1C levels include	Any condition that shortens the lifespan of a red blood cell will influence the hemoglobin A1C level. This includes: ❋ Hemolytic anemia	❋ Acute/chronic blood loss ❋ Sickle cell disease ❋ Pregnancy ❋ Chronic renal failure

Interfering Factors:

Falsely increased levels	Falsely decreased levels
• Falsely increased levels may be due to the presence of different sub-types of hemoglobin molecules e.g. hemoglobin F and uremia	• None noted

Related Tests:

Blood glucose, LDH

Triglycerides

Background

Triglycerides are composed primarily of fatty acid molecules attached to a glycerol backbone. They enter the blood stream endogenously from the liver and exogenously from the diet.

Exogenous sources of triglycerides:

In the digestive tract dietary fat, which is mostly triglyceride, is emulsified and broken down by pancreatic lipase into its constituent free fatty acids. These enter the intestinal mucosal cells and are re-formed into triglycerides that are incorporated into chylomicrons. The chylomicrons enter the bloodstream via the lymphatic lacteals and are cleared from the blood by tissue lipoprotein lipase, which breaks the triglycerides down into free fatty acids and glycerol. The free fatty acids are used for energy by the heart and skeletal muscle. They are also transported to the liver bound to albumin and/or reformed into triglycerides to be stored in adipose tissue.

Endogenous sources of triglycerides:

Endogenous sources of triglycerides come primarily from the liver, which synthesizes triglycerides from free fatty acids and glycerol.

Discussion

 Serum triglyceride levels are very much influenced by dietary fat consumption. Non-fasting samples are often the source of elevated triglycerides. A 12-hour fast is recommended to prevent the influence of dietary intake of fat on the sample. Post-prandial levels of triglycerides begin to rise about 2 hours after a meal, peaking at 4-6 hours.

- Patients that are metabolizing their fats and carbohydrates correctly tend to have a triglyceride level about one-half of the total cholesterol level. If the total cholesterol is 220, the triglycerides, in an ideal situation, should be about 110.

- Patients with abnormally elevated triglycerides and cholesterol level should be followed up with lipid electrophoresis, which is one of the best methods of assessing the metabolic problems associated with abnormal serum lipid values.

Ranges:

	Standard U.S. Units	Standard International Units
Conventional Laboratory Range	30 – 150 mg/dl	0.34 – 1.7 mmol/L
Optimal Range	70 – 110 mg/dl	0.79 – 1.24 mmol/L
Alarm Ranges	<35 or > 350 mg/dl	< 0.39 or > 3.95 mmol/L

When would you run this test?

1. As part of a cardiovascular screening assessment
2. As part of a lipid screening assessment
3. To monitor treatment
4. As part of a liver function study
5. As part of a thyroid function study

Clinical implications

HIGH

Clinical Implication	Additional information
Metabolic Syndrome /hyperinsulinemia	**Pattern:** If triglycerides are increased above the total cholesterol level with increased LDL cholesterol (>120 or 3.1 mmol/L), a decreased HDL (< 55 or < 1.42 mmol/L), and increased fasting blood glucose (> 100 or 5.55 mmol/L), then metabolic syndrome and hyperinsulinemia is **probable**. Metabolic Syndrome can lead to adrenal dysregulation, so adrenal stress should be ruled out. A diet high in refined sugars can cause the liver to produce excess triglycerides from carbohydrates and cause fatty acids to mobilize from the adipose tissue. In these situations the plasma levels of triglycerides increase beyond the body's capacity to clear them. This is a common pattern seen in cases of dysinsulinism and metabolic syndrome. Patients with this pattern will often do well on a low carbohydrate/high protein diet, especially the overweight and obese patients. **Please see the special topic on Metabolic Syndrome on page 9 for more details.**

Fatty liver (early development) and Liver congestion	Increased triglycerides are associated with liver congestion and the early development of fatty liver (steatosis). Fatty liver is caused by obesity, excessive alcohol consumption, prescription drugs (e.g. steroids), iron overload, solvent exposure, and rapid weight loss. Fatty changes to the liver tissue can impair the liver's detoxification ability. The degree of fatty liver changes is directly related to the amount of obesity. **Pattern:** If total cholesterol (>220 or 5.69 mmol/L), LDL (>120 or 3.1 mmol/L) and triglyceride levels (>110 or >1.24 mmol/L) are increased, and HDL levels are decreased (< 55 or < 1.42 mmol/L), then the early development of fatty liver is **possible**. Liver congestion, due to the fatty liver, should be considered if total cholesterol is above 220, triglycerides are increased (>110 or >1.24 mmol/L), and the SGPT/ALT is below 10. Fatty liver and liver congestion increases the risk of insulin resistance, hypertension, Metabolic Syndrome, and type II diabetes mellitus.
Early stage of insulin resistance	Elevated triglycerides often accompany the elevated glucose levels that are seen in insulin resistance.
Cardiovascular disease	Patients with a triglyceride level that is higher than the total cholesterol level and a decreased HDL (< 55 or < 1.42 mmol/L) have a higher risk for developing cardiovascular disease.
Atherosclerosis	An increased triglyceride level is associated with the development of atherosclerosis. Oxidative stress plays a large role in the process of cardiovascular disease. Over ¾ of patients with heart disease and high triglycerides will present with elevated levels of uric acid. Atherosclerosis is particularly accelerated in individuals with increased oxidative stress, a clinical presentation of metabolic syndrome, B-vitamin metabolism problems, increased homocysteine levels and familial hyperlipidemia. **Pattern:** If there is an increased triglyceride levels (>200 or 2.26

	mmol/L) in relation to total cholesterol (>220 or 5.69 mmol/L) with an increased uric acid level (>5.9 or > 351 μmol/dL), a decreased HDL (< 45 or < 1.16 mmol/L) and an increased LDL (>120 or 3.1 mmol/L), atherosclerosis is **probable**. Platelet levels may also be increased (>385). Homocysteine levels are frequently increased with atherosclerosis. Diabetes and thyroid hypofunction should also be considered with this pattern.
Poor metabolism and utilization of fats	This is often the case in patients that are eating an optimal diet and have elevated triglyceride and cholesterol levels.
Early stage of Hyperglycemia/Diabetes	Elevated triglycerides are seen in patients with diabetes. The triglycerides are often higher than the total cholesterol level. Lipid metabolism problems are a hallmark of the early stages of diabetes.
Hyperlipidemia	If HDL is less than 25% of the total cholesterol, then there is a strong clinical indication that hyperlipidemia is present. If the serum triglycerides and LDL are also increased, hyperlipidemia is likely present.
Primary hypothyroidism	Primary hypothyroidism is **possible** if the triglycerides and cholesterol levels are increased along with an increased TSH.
Adrenal cortical dysfunction	Consider adrenal cortical dysfunction if triglycerides and cholesterol levels are elevated with a decreased serum potassium. Catecholamines released from the adrenals can cause an increased release of fatty acids into the blood stream. Elevated cholesterol and other blood lipids increase with stress. Confirm with salivary adrenal studies or other functional adrenal tests.
Secondary Hypothyroidism **(Anterior pituitary hypofunction)**	An increased triglyceride levels is associated with secondary hypothyroidism due to an anterior pituitary dysfunction. **Pattern:** If triglyceride levels are increased (>110 or >1.24 mmol/L) with a decreased TSH (<2.0), then consider that anterior pituitary hypofunction is **probable**. If serum cholesterol is also elevated (>220 or 5.69 mmol/L), then thyroid hypofunction secondary to anterior pituitary hypofunction is **probable**. Some of the subjective indicators include: 1. Decreased libido

	2. Weight gain around hips or waist
	3. Menstrual irregularities
	4. Delayed sexual development (after age 13)
	5. Unresponsive thyroid treatment
	6. Hypoglycemia due to concomitant adrenal insufficiency

Diet and Serum Triglycerides

It is important to remember the following:

1. Elevated or decreased triglycerides alone are almost never the problem.

2. Elevated dietary fat is almost never the sole cause of elevated serum triglycerides.

Elevated serum triglycerides reflect a breakdown in the body's regulatory capacity and are more associated with blood sugar dysregulation in conjunction with dietary problems. It is important to review dietary patterns whenever patients present with elevated cholesterol and triglycerides. Review carbohydrate, alcohol, hydrogenated oil, and dairy intake. A diet high in carbohydrates and hydrogenated fats may cause an increase in serum triglycerides. Consider looking at some of the fundamental issues of fatty acid metabolism (liver, thyroid, blood sugar regulation, etc.) before rushing in with "green" supplements to lower cholesterol (niacin, garlic, gugulipid, etc.). It is a good idea to restrict the intake of grains and other foods high in starch, refined carbohydrates, fruit juices, alcohol, high glycemic fruits and vegetables, and hydrogenated oils.

Serum triglyceride clearance is accomplished by both the liver and muscle tissue. An effective method of reducing elevated triglyceride levels is to increase muscle demand for energy with vigorous cardiovascular exercise and/or resistance training.

| **Hyperlipoproteinemia** | Lipoprotein disorders usually present with elevated total cholesterol and triglyceride levels. There are 6 distinctive sub-types of these disorders, which are mostly genetic in nature. The lipid electrophoresis is one of the bests methods for determining the various metabolic problems associated with hyperlipoproteinemia. |

Alcoholism	Alcohol is extremely calorie dense. Regular alcohol consumption and alcoholism can lead to significantly elevated levels of triglycerides in the blood. This is often accompanied by a greatly increased GGTP.	
Drug causes of ⬆	Drugs can affect lipid levels in a number of different ways. The toxic effects of most drugs can interfere with lipid synthesis.	
	✳ Beta-blockers	✳ Diuretics
	✳ Cholestyramine	✳ Estrogens
	✳ Corticosteroids	✳ Oral contraceptives
	✳ Diazepam	
Other conditions associated with increased triglyceride levels include	✳ Diabetes	✳ Viral hepatitis
	✳ Acute pancreatitis	✳ Glycogen storage diseases
	✳ Nephritic syndrome	✳ Anorexia
	✳ Gout and uremia	

LOW

Clinical Implication	Additional information
Liver/biliary dysfunction	Biliary congestion can impact on the emulsification and digestion of fats, which may lead to a decreased level of triglycerides. Liver dysfunction, such as fatty liver, can also prevent the synthesis of endogenous triglycerides and other lipids and lipoproteins.
Diet- Nutrient deficient, insufficient fat intake, vegetarian diet	Dietary intake of healthy fats maybe low, a pattern that is commonly seen in vegetarians.
Thyroid hyperfunction	Hyperthyroidism is **probable** if there are low triglycerides (<70 or <0.79 mmol/L) with a low TSH (<2.0) and a high T-3 (>230 or 3.53 nmol/L), T-3 uptake (>37), T-4 (>12 or 154.4 nmol/L), and/or FTI. The low triglyceride levels are probably due to the excessive utilization of fatty acids by a metabolism that is excessively fast.
Autoimmune processes	If triglycerides are decreased (<40 or 0.45 mmol/L) with low or normal cholesterol (160 – 220 or 4.14 – 5.69 mmol/L) and an increased HDL (>70 or 1.81 mmol/L), then some kind of

	autoimmune process in the body is **possible**. The problem may be inflammatory or destructive in nature. Consider further testing to rule-out tissue inflammation or destruction (C-reactive protein, ANA, rheumatoid factor etc.). If tissue destruction is present, LDH, Alpha 1 or Alpha 2 globulin (seen with serum protein electrophoresis) will frequently be increased. This may also be a sign of endocrine dysfunction due to endocrine hypo or hyper function. Consider further endocrine testing to locate cause of the disturbance.
Adrenal hyperfunction	Low triglyceride levels may be due to the excessive metabolism often seen in adrenal hyperfunction.
Drug causes of ↓	✳ Clofibrate ✳ Nicotinic acid ✳ Gemfibrizol

Other conditions associated with decreased triglyceride levels include	🌰 Endurance exercise 🌰 Excessive oxidative stress 🌰 Free radical pathology	🌰 Chemical or heavy metal overload 🌰 Digestive dysfunction/ malabsorption

Interfering Factors:

Increased bilirubin, uric acid or vitamin C can interfere with accurate triglyceride results

Falsely increased levels	**Falsely decreased levels**
• High fat diet, alcohol intake, pregnancy, obesity, severe acute stress • High alkaline phosphatase levels will increase triglyceride levels to some degree	• Ascorbic acid

Related Tests:

Total cholesterol, LDL, HDL, lipoprotein studies, blood glucose, lipid electrophoresis, serum homocysteine, Oxidata free radical test

Cholesterol

Background

Cholesterol is a steroid found in every cell of the body and in the plasma. It is an essential component in the structure of the cell membrane where it controls membrane fluidity. It provides the structural backbone for every steroid hormone in the body, which includes adrenal and sex hormones and vitamin D. The myelin sheaths of nerve fibers are derived from cholesterol and the bile salts that emulsify fats are composed of cholesterol.

Cholesterol is derived from endogenous synthesis by the liver and other organs, and from exogenous dietary sources. The liver, the intestines, and the skin produce between 60-80% of the body's cholesterol. The remainder comes from the diet.

Discussion

The link between cholesterol and cardiovascular disease is widely known, yet is not as important. What are not so well recognized are cholesterol's antioxidant activities in the body.

- Cholesterol, in its unoxidized form, has free radical scavenging properties, and as such functions as a natural cell membrane protector. It protects cells from cancer and other free-radical induced diseases. Thus low levels of cholesterol present an increased risk for oxidative stress. In its oxidized state, cholesterol can act as a pro-oxidant and a free radical producer.

- Cholesterol is synthesized from acetyl-CoA in a series of enzymatic steps that require vitamins B6, B12, and folate as coenzymes. Cholesterol synthesis shares its rate-limiting enzyme HMG-CoA reductase with the enzymatic synthesis of Coenzyme Q10.

 HMG-CoA reductase is the target of many of the cholesterol lowering drugs, whose activity can play havoc on the body's synthesis of CoQ-10.

- Total cholesterol comprises all of the cholesterol found in the body, i.e. LDL cholesterol, HDL cholesterol, and triglycerides/5, which is an estimation of VLDL cholesterol. Levels are influenced by metabolic rate, and increased levels of cholesterol are often associated with thyroid or adrenal hypofunction. Conversely, decreased levels are associated with endocrine hyperfunction.

- Although total serum cholesterol can give a good general assessment of cardiovascular risk, other tests and markers should be taken into consideration to give a more accurate and complete picture of possible atherosclerotic coronary artery disease risk. These include apolipoprotein A and B, HDL, LDL, VLDL, serum homocysteine, and triglycerides.

Note:

Cholesterol values should only be taken after at least a 12-hour fast.

Ranges:

	Standard U.S. Units	Standard International Units
Conventional Laboratory Range	130 – 200 mg/dL	3.36 – 5.2 mmol/L
Optimal Range	150 – 220 mg/dL	3.9 – 5.69 mmol/L
Alarm Ranges	<50 or > 400 mg/dL	<1.29 or > 10.34 mmol/L

When would you run this test?

1. As part of a lipid screening assessment
2. To monitor treatment
3. As part of a liver function study
4. As part of a thyroid function study

Clinical implications

HIGH

Clinical Implication	Additional information
Primary hypothyroidism	Primary hypothyroidism is **possible** if the total cholesterol is increased along with an increased triglyceride and TSH.
Adrenal cortical dysfunction	Consider adrenal cortical dysfunction if cholesterol is elevated with an increased triglyceride level and a decreased serum potassium. Catecholamines released from the adrenals can cause an increased release of fatty acids into the blood stream. Elevated cholesterol and other blood lipids increase with stress. Confirm with salivary adrenal studies or other functional adrenal tests.

Secondary Hypothyroidism **(Anterior pituitary hypofunction)**	Increased cholesterol levels are associated with thyroid hypofunction that is secondary to an anterior pituitary hypofunction. **Pattern:** If cholesterol levels are increased (>220 or 5.69 mmol/L) with a decreased TSH (<2.0), then consider that anterior pituitary hypofunction is **probable**. If serum triglycerides are also elevated (>110 or >1.24 mmol/L), then thyroid hypofunction secondary to anterior pituitary hypofunction is **probable**. Some of the subjective indicators include: 1. Decreased libido 2. Weight gain around hips or waist 3. Menstrual irregularities 4. Delayed sexual development (after age 13) 5. Unresponsive thyroid treatment 6. Hypoglycemia due to concomitant adrenal insufficiency
Cardiovascular disease	Patients with a triglyceride level that is higher than the total cholesterol level and a decreased HDL (< 55 or < 1.42 mmol/L) have a higher risk for developing cardiovascular disease.
Atherosclerosis	Increased cholesterol levels are associated with hyperlipidemia, which has been shown to indicate a potential risk of developing atherosclerotic coronary artery disease. Although this may be true, it is important to look at many of the other risks for this disease before jumping to conclusion that elevated cholesterol levels are the culprit. Other risks for atherosclerosis and cardiovascular disease include: smoking, elevated homocysteine levels, B6, B12 and folate deficiency, ingestion of chlorine, blood sugar dysregulation, and hypertension. **Pattern:** If there is an increased triglyceride level (>200 or 2.26 mmol/L) in relation to total cholesterol (>220 or 5.69 mmol/L) with an increased uric acid level (>5.9 or > 351 µmol/dL), a decreased HDL (<45 or 1.16 mmol/L) and an increased LDL (>120 or 3.1 mmol/L), atherosclerosis is

	probable. Platelet (> 385) and Homocysteine levels are frequently increased with atherosclerosis.
Biliary stasis	Thickened bile is the hallmark of biliary stasis. It may occur if the total cholesterol is increased (>220 or 5.69 mmol/L). This may be the only finding on the chem. screen i.e. normal GGTP, SGPT/ALT, and bilirubin. The subjective findings in biliary stasis include: 1. Strong craving for sweets 2. Nausea 3. Gallbladder attacks (past or present) 4. Headache over the eye 5. Bitter taste in the mouth 6. Greasy or high fat foods cause distress 7. Pain between shoulder blades 8. Light brown or yellow stools
Early stage of insulin resistance	Elevated cholesterol and other lipids often accompany the elevated glucose levels that are seen in insulin resistance.
Poor metabolism and utilization of fats	This is often the case in patients that are eating an optimal diet and have elevated cholesterol and triglyceride levels.
Fatty liver (early development) and Liver congestion	If total cholesterol (>220 or 5.69 mmol/L), LDL (>120 or 3.1 mmol/L) and triglyceride levels (>110 or >1.24 mmol/L) are increased, and HDL levels are decreased (< 55 or < 1.42 mmol/L), then the early development of fatty liver is **possible**. Liver congestion, due to the fatty liver, should be considered if total cholesterol is above 220 or 5.69 mol/L, triglycerides are increased (>110 or >1.24 mmol/L), and the SGPT/ALT is below 10. Fatty liver is caused by obesity, excessive alcohol consumption, prescription drugs (e.g. steroids), iron overload, solvent exposure, and rapid weight loss. Fatty changes to the liver tissue can impair the liver's detoxification ability. The degree of fatty liver changes is directly related to the amount of obesity. Fatty liver and liver congestion increases the risk of insulin resistance, hypertension, Metabolic Syndrome, and type II diabetes mellitus.
Early stage of Hyperglycemia/Diabetes	Elevated blood lipids are seen in patients with diabetes. The triglycerides are often higher than the total cholesterol level. Lipid metabolism problems are a hallmark of the early stages of diabetes.

Metabolic Syndrome /hyperinsulinemia	**Pattern:** If triglycerides are increased above the total cholesterol level with increased LDL cholesterol (>120 or 3.1 mmol/L), a decreased HDL (< 55 or < 1.42 mmol/L), and increased fasting blood glucose (> 100 or 5.55 mmol/L), then metabolic syndrome and hyperinsulinemia is **probable**. Metabolic Syndrome can lead to adrenal dysregulation, so adrenal stress should be ruled out. A diet high in refined sugars can cause the liver to produce excess triglycerides from carbohydrates and cause fatty acids to mobilize from the adipose tissue. In these situations the plasma levels of triglycerides increase beyond the body's capacity to clear them. This is a common pattern seen in cases of dysinsulinism and metabolic syndrome. Patients with this pattern will often do well on a low carbohydrate/high protein diet, especially the overweight and obese patients. **Please see the special topic on Metabolic Syndrome on page 9 for more details.**

Diet and Cholesterol

Focusing on just lowering dietary cholesterol and fat consumption usually has little to no effect on serum cholesterol levels. A diet high in carbohydrates, especially refined carbohydrates, starches, and other fast acting sugars and hydrogenated fats is more likely to cause an increase in total cholesterol. The greatest effect on lowering serum cholesterol levels will be made by addressing other factors such as excessive carbohydrate consumption, sedentary lifestyle, smoking, endocrine dysfunction, and liver/biliary congestion.

Hyperlipoproteinemia	Lipoprotein disorders usually present with elevated total cholesterol and triglyceride levels. There are 6 distinctive sub-types of these disorders, which are mostly genetic in nature. The lipid electrophoresis is one of the best methods for determining the various metabolic problems associated with hyperlipoproteinemia.
Multiple sclerosis	Multiple sclerosis presents with variable findings on blood chemistries. Frequently the total cholesterol will be increased along with a decreased Alkaline Phosphatase intestinal isoenzyme. MS is associated with the following factors:

	• Genetic predisposition	
	• Heavy metal body burden	
	• Intestinal/systemic parasites	
	• Bacterial or viral infections	
	• Exposure to chemicals	
	MS is also strongly associated with gluten insensitivity and an inability to correctly and adequately metabolize the trans fatty acids in hydrogenated fats. All sources should be removed from their diets.	
Other conditions associated with increased levels include	✳ Pregnancy ✳ Type II familial hypercholesterolemia ✳ Hyperlipoproteinemia	✳ Nephritic syndrome ✳ Pancreatic and prostatic malignant neoplasms ✳ Alcoholism

LOW

Clinical Implication	Additional information
Oxidative Stress and Free Radical Activity	Suspect excess free radical activity and oxidative stress if the total cholesterol is suddenly below its historical level. **Pattern:** If a total cholesterol level is suddenly below its historical level and is seen with a decreased lymphocyte count (<20), a decreased albumin (<4.0 or 40g/L) and platelet level (<150), an increased total globulin (>2.8 or 28 g/L) and uric acid level (>5.9 or > 351 µmol/dL), free radical pathology, which increases the risk for developing a neoplasm, should be investigated. This can be accomplished in the office using the Oxidata free radical test. **Please see page 152 for a discussion of this test.** Oxidative stress can cause an increased destruction of red blood cells; in these situations you will see an elevated bilirubin level. **Other tests include**: Acid Phosphatase, serum protein Electrophoresis, CEA, Anti-malignin Antibody, HCG, Alpha Fetoprotein, etc. If Alpha 1, Alpha 2, or gamma globulins are increased on a serum protein electrophoresis, free radical pathology should be investigated immediately. Unoxidized cholesterol acts as an antioxidant in the body, so decreased levels put the body at risk for developing oxidative stress, especially lipid peroxidation, and increases the chance of free radical induced diseases.

Decreased cholesterol levels- as bad as elevated levels?

It is well known that elevated cholesterol levels pose an increased risk for developing atherosclerotic coronary artery disease. What is not so well known is that a decreased cholesterol level can be just as harmful. Cholesterol provides the structure for the following:

1. Cellular membranes, where it helps regulate membrane fluidity and intra-cellular communication

2. Myelin sheaths, where it provides for the structure of the myelin sheaths in the nervous system, which helps regulate nerve transmission

3. Steroid hormones, where it provides the backbone for adrenal hormones, sex hormones, and vitamin D.

Harry Eidenier, PhD, using electrophoretic studies, hormonal studies, glycoprotein electrophoresis, CBC with differential and other blood studies, was able to confirm that a sudden decreased cholesterol for a patient who historically had not had low cholesterol, was a strong diagnostic indicator of an increased oxidative stress and potential neoplastic development.

Decreased levels of cholesterol may lead to nervous system dysfunction and poor hormonal synthesis, as well as increased levels of stress to the cardiovascular system. The immune system, which relies heavily on cellular communication and recognition, may be at a great risk too. Given the above list of essential functions of cholesterol to the human metabolism, it is not difficult to see why low cholesterol is as dangerous as high.

Heavy metal/Chemical overload	Patients with historically low total cholesterol levels may be more prone to heavy metal and chemical toxins due to poor cell membrane integrity. This is irrespective of level of exposure, but related more to susceptibility of the individual patient. This may also leave patients at an increased risk for developing neoplasm.
Liver/biliary dysfunction	Biliary congestion can lead to a dysfunctional gallbladder, which can impact the emulsification and digestion of fats, potentially leading to a decreased level of cholesterol. Liver dysfunction, such as late stage fatty liver, can also prevent the synthesis of endogenous cholesterol, triglycerides, and other lipids and lipoproteins.

	J. Mercola, DO, in his newsletter "Healthy News you can use", http://www.mercola.com, reported that, in his opinion, most low cholesterol levels are due to a dysfunctional gallbladder.
Diet- Malnutrition (insufficient fat intake, vegetarian diet)	Low cholesterol is a pattern that is commonly seen in vegetarians. The dietary intake of healthy fats is low. Check red blood cell levels of essential fatty acids to determine essential fatty acid need.
Thyroid hyperfunction	Hyperthyroidism is **probable** with low triglycerides (<70 or <0.79 mmol/L) with a low TSH (<2.0) and a high T-3 (>230 or 3.53 nmol/L), T-3 uptake (>37), T-4 (>12 or 154.4), and/or FTI. The low cholesterol levels may be due to the excessive utilization of fatty acids by a metabolism that is excessively fast.

To receive master copies of our tracking forms and conversion tables please visit:

www.BloodChemistryAnalysis.com

If you're interested in a software program to help with your analysis please visit:
www.BloodChemSoftware.com

Autoimmune processes	If the cholesterol level is low or normal (160-220 or 4.14-5.69 mmol/L), triglycerides are decreased (<40 or 0.45 mmol/L) and HDL is increased (>70 or 1.81 mmol/L), then some kind of autoimmune process in the body is **possible**. The problem may be inflammatory or destructive in nature. Consider further testing to rule out tissue inflammation or destruction (C-reactive protein, ANA, rheumatoid factor etc.). If tissue destruction is present, LDH, Alpha 1, or Alpha 2 globulin (seen with serum protein electrophoresis) will frequently be increased.
	This may also be a sign of endocrine dysfunction due to endocrine hypo or hyper function. Consider further endocrine testing to locate cause of the disturbance.
Adrenal hyperfunction	Low cholesterol levels may be due to the excessive metabolism often seen in patients with adrenal hyperfunction. They are burning up their lipids with their high levels of hormones.

Other conditions associated with decreased total cholesterol levels include	🫀 Digestive dysfunction/ malabsorption ⚕ Severe liver disease (acute viral hepatitis, malignant liver neoplasm, cirrhosis)	⚕ Severe burns ⚕ COPD 🫀 Megaloblastic anemia

Interfering Factors:

Falsely increased levels	Falsely decreased levels
• Thiazide diuretic therapy increases cholesterol levels by much as 5-8% • Levels tend to be higher in the fall and winter	• Values may decrease by as much as 10% when a patient changes from a standing to a recumbent position • Major illnesses can decrease cholesterol levels e.g. post MI, bacterial sepsis and viral infections • High ascorbic acid levels • Levels tend to be lower in the spring and summer

Related Tests:

Apolipoprotein A and B, HDL, LDL, VLDL, triglycerides, lipid electrophoresis, Serum homocysteine, Oxidata Free Radical Test

LDL

Discussion

LDL contains most of the cholesterol in the serum and is the lipoprotein that carries the majority of the essential fatty acids from the liver to the tissue. LDL levels are inversely related to HDL in terms of their ratios. As LDL increases, HDL levels decrease and vise versa. LDL has a better correlation with risk of atherosclerosis than total cholesterol. There is also an association between increased LDL levels coupled with decreased HDL levels and an increased risk of atherosclerotic coronary artery disease, diabetes, and metabolic syndrome.

- LDL functions to transport cholesterol and other fatty acids from the liver to the peripheral tissues for uptake and metabolism by the cells. It is known as "bad cholesterol" because it is thought that this process of bringing cholesterol from the liver to the peripheral tissue increases the risk for atherosclerosis.

LDL- a calculated measurement

LDL is a calculated measurement. Most lab panels do not provide actual measurements of LDL. The LDL fraction is estimated from the following formula:

LDL cholesterol = Total cholesterol – (HDL + Triglycerides/5).

Total cholesterol is composed of LDL, HDL and VLDL cholesterol. Triglycerides/5 is an estimation of the VLDL portion of the total cholesterol, since the majority of the plasma triglyceride is in the VLDL portion.

- This is a fairly accurate assessment, though there have been those that recommend that triglycerides be divided by 6 to give an even more accurate estimation of LDL.

- The one problem with using this formula is that it is based on three different tests. One or more inaccurate test results can seriously affect the LDL calculation.

- In addition, the formula cannot be used when triglyceride levels are greater than 400 mg/dL (>4.52 mmol/L). In this case a direct determination of LDL is needed.

Ranges:

	Standard U.S. Units	Standard International Units
Conventional Laboratory Range	60 – 130 mg/dL	1.55 – 3.36 mmol/L
Optimal Range	<120 mg/dL	< 3.10 mmol/L
Alarm Ranges	> 200 mg/dL	> 5.17 mmol/L

When would you run this test?

1. As part of a cardiovascular screening assessment

2. As part of a lipid screening assessment

3. To screen for Metabolic Syndrome and blood sugar dysregulation

4. To monitor treatment

5. As part of a liver or thyroid function study

Clinical implications

HIGH

Clinical Implication	Additional information
Diet- high in refined carbohydrates	The Standard American Diet (SAD), which is very high in refined carbohydrates, can contribute to increased LDL
Metabolic Syndrome /hyperinsulinemia	If LDL levels are increased (>120 or 3.1 mmol/L), triglycerides are increased above the total cholesterol level with decreased HDL cholesterol (< 55 or < 1.42 mmol/L), and increased fasting blood glucose (> 100 or 5.55 mmol/L), then metabolic syndrome and hyperinsulinemia is **probable**. Metabolic Syndrome can lead to adrenal dysregulation, so adrenal hyperfunctioning should be ruled out. **Please see the special topic on Metabolic Syndrome on page 9 for more details.**
Atherosclerosis	An increased LDL level is associated with the development of atherosclerosis. Oxidative stress plays a large role in the process of cardiovascular disease. Over ¾ of patients with heart disease and high triglycerides will present with elevated levels of uric acid. Atherosclerosis is particularly accelerated in individuals with

	increased oxidative stress, a clinical presentation of metabolic syndrome, B-vitamin metabolism problems, increased homocysteine levels, and familial hyperlipidemia. **Pattern:** If there is an increased triglyceride levels (>200 or 2.26 mmol/L) in relation to total cholesterol (>220 or 5.69 mmol/L) with an increased uric acid level (>5.9 or > 351 μmol/dL), a decreased HDL (<45 or 1.16 mmol/L), and an increased LDL (>120 or 3.1 mmol/L), atherosclerosis is **probable**. Platelet levels may also be increased (>385). Homocysteine levels are frequently increased with atherosclerosis. Diabetes and thyroid hypofunction should also be considered with this pattern.
Hyperlipidemia	Increased LDL cholesterol and total cholesterol levels are associated with hyperlipidemia, which has been shown to indicate a potential risk of developing atherosclerotic coronary artery disease. **Pattern:** If LDL is increased (>120 or 3.1 mmol/L) with an increased total cholesterol (>220 or 5.69 mmol/L) and LDL/HDL ratio and an increased level of triglycerides (>110 or >1.24 mmol/L) with HDL less than 25% of the total cholesterol, hyperlipidemia is **probable.**
Oxidative stress	Increased LDL levels are associated with increasing free radical activity and oxidative stress. The peroxidation of LDL may promote the accumulation of cholesterol in the macrophages and smooth muscle cells, which can lead to atherosclerotic plaque formation.
Fatty liver (early development) and Liver congestion	If LDL levels are increased, along with increased triglyceride and total cholesterol levels, and HDL levels are decreased, the early development of fatty liver is **possible**. Liver congestion, due to the fatty liver, should be considered if total cholesterol is above 220 or 5.69 mmol/L, triglycerides are increased (>110 or >1.24 mmol/L), and the SGPT/ALT is below 10. Fatty liver is caused by obesity, excessive alcohol consumption, prescription drugs (e.g. steroids), iron overload, solvent exposure, and rapid weight loss. Fatty changes to the liver tissue can impair the liver's detoxification ability. The degree of fatty liver changes is directly related to the amount

	of obesity.	
	Fatty liver and liver congestion increase the risk of insulin resistance, hypertension, Metabolic Syndrome, and type II diabetes mellitus.	
Drug causes of ↑	❅ Estrogen ❅ Progestins ❅ Birth Control Pills ❅ Androgens	
Other conditions associated with increased LDL levels include	🖐 Heavy metal/Chemical overload 🖐 Hypothyroidism 🖐 ↑ Saturated fat diet ❅ Nephritic syndrome ❅ Familial type II Hypercholesterolemia	❅ Multiple myeloma ❅ Hepatic obstruction ❅ Anorexia nervosa ❅ Diabetes mellitus ❅ Chronic renal failure

Interfering Factors:

Falsely increased levels	Falsely decreased levels
• Pregnancy	• None noted

Related Tests:

Total cholesterol, HDL, triglycerides, lipoprotein studies, blood glucose, lipid electrophoresis, serum homocysteine, Oxidata free radical test and Uric acid, RBC, HCT and HGB (will often be increased with developing atherosclerotic condition)

HDL

Background

Lipoproteins are molecules that are composed of lipids (triglycerides, cholesterol, phospholipids) and proteins (apoprotein) in various proportions. The High Density Lipoprotein, also known as HDL, is composed of primarily phospholipid and apoproteins in its structure. HDL functions to transport cholesterol from the peripheral tissues and vessel walls to the liver for processing and metabolism into bile salts. It is known as "good cholesterol" because it is thought that this process of bringing cholesterol from the peripheral tissue to the liver is protective against atherosclerosis. Further protective benefits of HDL may be due to its ability to influence the absorption and binding of LDL by smooth muscle and other cells.

Discussion

 HDL must be viewed in relation to the total cholesterol and the LDL cholesterol levels. If the total cholesterol is low, a decreased HDL level is not considered a cardiovascular risk. If the total cholesterol is elevated, HDL can be used as a strong independent diagnostic indicator to determine the risk for atherosclerotic coronary artery disease.

- Decreased HDL is considered atherogenic, increased HDL is considered protective. Both HDL and total cholesterol are independent risk factors.

- It is quite common for one value to be normal and the other value to be elevated; a value that has a favorable effect does not entirely cancel the unfavorable effect of the other.

Ranges:

	Standard U.S. Units	Standard International Units
Conventional Laboratory Range	40 – 90 mg/dL	1.03 – 2.32 mmol/L
Optimal Range	> 55 mg/dL	> 1.42 mmol/L
Alarm Ranges	< 35 mg/dL	< 0.91 mmol/L

When would you run this test?

1. As part of a cardiovascular risk assessment
2. As part of a lipid screening assessment
3. To screen for metabolic syndrome and blood sugar dysregulation
4. To monitor treatment
5. As part of a liver and thyroid function study

Clinical implications

HIGH

Clinical Implication	Additional information	
Autoimmune processes	If HDL cholesterol is increased (>70 or 1.81 mmol/L), and triglycerides are decreased (<40 or 0.45 mmol/L) with low or normal cholesterol (160-220 or 4.13-5.69 mmol/L), then some kind of autoimmune process in the body is **possible**. The problem may be inflammatory or destructive in nature. Consider further testing to rule-out tissue inflammation or destruction (C-reactive protein, ANA, rheumatoid factor etc.). If tissue destruction is present, LDH, Alpha 1 or Alpha 2 globulin (seen with serum protein electrophoresis) will frequently be increased.	
	This may also be a sign of endocrine dysfunction due to endocrine hypo or hyper function. Consider further endocrine testing to locate the cause of the disturbance.	
	Before running these tests ask the patient about historical HDL levels, whether they have a genetic predisposition i.e. family history, or whether they are exercising heavily. These factors may contribute to significantly increased HDL levels in a healthy patient.	
Drug causes of ↑	❈ Estrogen ❈ Estrogen in combination with androgens ❈ Steroids	
Other conditions associated with increased HDL levels include	❈ Hypothyroidism ❈ Insulin use	❈ Exogenous estrogen ❈ Excessive alcohol consumption

LOW

Clinical Implication	Additional information
Hyperlipidemia and atherosclerosis	If HDL is less than 25% of the total cholesterol, then there is a strong clinical indication that hyperlipidemia is present. If the serum triglycerides (>110 or >1.24 mmol/L) and LDL (>120 or 3.1 mmol/L) are also increased, hyperlipidemia is likely present and atherosclerosis should be ruled-out.
Diets high in refined carbohydrates	The Standard American Diet (SAD), which is very high in refined carbohydrates, can contribute to decreased HDL levels (< 55 or < 1.42 mmol/L)
Metabolic Syndrome /hyperinsulinemia	**Pattern:** If HDL levels are decreased (< 55 or < 1.42 mmol/L), triglycerides are increased above the total cholesterol level with increased LDL cholesterol (>120 or 3.1 mmol/L) and increased fasting blood glucose (> 100 or 5.55 mmol/L), then Metabolic Syndrome and hyperinsulinemia are **probable**. Metabolic Syndrome can lead to adrenal dysregulation, so adrenal hyperfunctioning should be ruled out. **Please see the special topic on Metabolic Syndrome on page 9 for more details.**
Oxidative stress	Unoxidized cholesterol, including HDL cholesterol, acts as an antioxidant and a free radical scavenger in the body, so decreased levels put the body at risk for developing oxidative stress, especially lipid peroxidation, and increases the chance of free radical induced diseases.
Heavy metal/Chemical overload	Patients with historically low HDL and total cholesterol levels may be more prone to heavy metal and chemical toxins due to poor cell membrane integrity. This is irrespective of level of exposure, but related more to susceptibility of the individual patient. This may also leave patients at an increased risk for developing neoplasm.
Fatty liver (early development) and Liver congestion	If HDL levels are decreased (< 55 or < 1.42 mmol/L), and LDL (>120 or 3.1 mmol/L), triglyceride (>110 or >1.24 mmol/L) and total cholesterol levels (>220 or 5.69 mmol/L) are increased, then the early development of fatty liver is **possible**. Liver congestion, due to the fatty liver, should be considered if total cholesterol is above 220 or 5.69 mmol/L, triglycerides are increased (>110 or >1.24 mmol/L), and the SGPT/ALT is below 10. Fatty liver is caused by obesity, excessive alcohol

	consumption, prescription drugs (e.g. steroids), iron overload, solvent exposure, and rapid weight loss. Fatty changes to the liver tissue can impair the liver's detoxification ability. The degree of fatty liver changes is directly related to the amount of obesity. Fatty liver and liver congestion increases the risk of insulin resistance, hypertension, Metabolic Syndrome, and type II diabetes mellitus.
Hyperthyroidism	The increased metabolic activity found in hyperthyroidism can lead to decreased HDL levels. The body preferentially uses fatty acids, which are transported via lipoproteins, for energy in this heightened metabolic state.
Lack of exercise/ sedentary lifestyle	A sedentary lifestyle has been shown to decrease HDL levels. Increasing cardiovascular and resistance exercise is a very good way to elevate HDL levels.
Drug causes of ↓	✾ Thiazide diuretics ✾ Antihypertensive medications ✾ Beta blockers without sympathomimetic activity ✾ Sympatholytic agents

Other conditions associated with decreased HDL levels include	✾ Obesity ✾ Genetic predisposition	✾ Starvation ✾ Uremia

Interfering Factors:

Falsely increased levels	Falsely decreased levels
• None noted	• Ascorbic acid may cause a 5-15% decrease in HDL levels • Temporary decrease after MI

Related Tests:

Total cholesterol, LDL, triglycerides, lipoprotein studies, blood glucose, lipid electrophoresis, serum homocysteine, Oxidata free radical test, RBC, HCT and HGB (will often be increased with developing atherosclerotic condition)

Apolipoprotein A and B

Background

Apolipoproteins are a protein component of lipoprotein complexes. Apolipoprotein A-1 is the major component of HDL and Apolipoprotein B is the major component of LDL

Discussion

Elevated levels of apolipoprotein A-1 are believed to be a greater predictor for lower incidence of cardiovascular disease than HDL alone. Studies have shown that Apolipoprotein A-1 is the best predictor of family history of myocardial infarction in young men.

Elevated levels of apolipoprotein B are associated with an increased risk of atherosclerotic coronary artery disease.

Some would suggest that Apolipoprotein A-1 and B are much better markers for cardiovascular disease than traditional lipid studies

Ranges:

	Standard U.S. Units	**Standard International Units**
Conventional Laboratory Range	**Apo A-1**: 110 – 162 mg/dL **Apo B**: 52 – 109 mg/dL	
Optimal Range	**Apo A-1**: 110 – 162 mg/dL **Apo B**: 52 – 109 mg/dL	

When would you run this test?

1. To gather more data on cardiovascular risk assessment

Clinical implications

HIGH

Clinical Implication	Additional information
Apolipoprotein A-1	Predictive of a lowered incidence of cardiovascular disease
Apolipoprotein B	Predictive of an increased incidence or premature coronary artery disease Also: diabetes, hypothyroidism, nephrotic syndrome, renal failure, Porphyria, Cushing's syndrome

LOW

Clinical Implication	Additional information
Apolipoprotein A-1	Associated with an increased incidence of premature cardiovascular disease Also: poorly controlled diabetes, hepatocellular disease, nephrotic syndrome, renal failure
Apolipoprotein B	Suggestive of a lowered incidence of cardiovascular disease Also: hypothyroidism, malnutrition, malabsorption, chronic anemias, Reye's syndrome, Acute stress, inflammatory joint disease

Interfering Factors:

Falsely increased levels	Falsely decreased levels
• Various prescription drugs can falsely elevate Apolipoprotein studies	• Apolipoprotein A-1: a diet high in polyunsaturated fats, smoking, androgens and oral contraceptive use • Apolipoprotein B: Diets high in polyunsaturated fats

Related Tests:

Triglycerides, cholesterol, LDL, HDL, VLDL, Uric acid, lipid electrophoresis, RBC, HCT and HGB (will often be increased with developing atherosclerotic condition)

BUN
Blood Urea Nitrogen

Background

Urea is formed in the liver and is the final product in protein catabolism, along with CO_2. It is formed almost entirely by the liver from both protein metabolism and protein digestion. BUN reflects the ratio between the production and clearance of urea. The amount of urea excreted as BUN varies with the amount of dietary protein intake. Increased BUN may be due to an increased production of urea by the liver or decreased excretion by the kidney.

Discussion

The BUN is a test that is predominantly used to measure kidney function. Unfortunately, when using blood chemistry analysis you can only make a judgment as to what is actually happening in the kidney itself and speculate at best to the etiology and severity of the problem. Further kidney testing must be performed to ascertain the nature of the problem.

- BUN is useful as a first indicator of renal insufficiency especially if all the other renal indicators are normal.

- Urea is removed almost entirely by the kidneys; however, a significant amount travels from the liver to the colon and is acted upon by gut microflora to recirculate nitrogen, making it a useful indicator for dysbiosis. In the large intestine, putrefactive action of increased bacterial overgrowth on nitrogenous materials releases significant quantities of ammonia. Some of this ammonia will be converted into urea by the liver leading to increased BUN levels.

Ranges:

	Standard U.S. Units	Standard International Units
Conventional Laboratory Range	5 – 25 mg/dL	1.79 – 8.93 mmol/L
Optimal Range	10 – 16 mg/dL	3.57 – 5.71 mmol/L
Alarm Ranges	< 5 mg/dL or	< 1.79 mmol/L or
	> 50 mg/dL	> 17.85 mmol/L

When would you run this test?

1. This test is useful to screen for renal insufficiency

2. This test is useful to assess liver dysfunction

3. To screen for functional digestive problems and for dehydration

Clinical implications

HIGH

Clinical Implication	Additional information
Renal disease 	The pattern found below is indicative of an impaired renal function, which should be ruled out and referred to a qualified practitioner if present. However, an elevated BUN found in isolation of the pattern below is more indicative of renal insufficiency or other causes. **Pattern:** Increased BUN (>25 or 8.93 mmol/L), serum creatinine (>1.4 or >123.8 µmol/dL), BUN/Creatinine ratio (10-20), Urine specific gravity (1.010 - 1.016), Uric acid (>5.9 or > 351 µmol/dL), serum phosphorous (>4.0 or 1.29 mmol/L) LDH (>200), and SGOT/AST (>30).
Renal insufficiency	An increased BUN level (>16 or 5.71 mmol/L) can be a sign of renal insufficiency. Renal insufficiency is an often over-looked condition. **Please see the special topic below for more details.** **Pattern:** Suspect renal insufficiency if there is an increased BUN level (>16 or 5.71 mmol/L) with a normal or increased serum Creatinine (>1.1 or 97.2µmol/dL), a normal to increased Uric Acid (>5.9 or > 351 µmol/dL), and an increased serum phosphorous (>4.0 or 1.29 mmol/L). LDH and SGOT/AST will usually be normal.

Renal Insufficiency

Renal insufficiency or decreased renal function occurs long before one sees overt renal disease. The kidneys help to filter waste and toxins, but this is not their only function. They regulate fluid and mineral balance, help regulate blood pressure, secrete hormones (erythropoietin, rennin, angiotensin, prostaglandins), and regulate acid-base balance amongst other functions. There are many factors that contribute to renal insufficiency.

- Heavy metal toxicity has a detrimental effect on kidney function. Cadmium and mercury, which slowly destroys the glomeruli, are especially deleterious.

- Factors that cause an increased stress on the kidneys include: high protein intake, processed foods, sugar, caffeine, alcohol etc.

- Many over the counter and prescription drugs cause damage to the kidney.

- Dehydration can cause a significant stress on the kidneys.

- Impaired liver function, especially its detoxification function can lead to increased kidney stress. The kidney will often take on many of the detoxification tasks of the liver when the liver becomes compromised.

- It is very common to have sub-acute, long-term low-grade and chronic idiopathic infections that will decrease kidney function over time.

In Chinese medicine the skin is associated with the kidney. The body will use the skin as a secondary route of detoxification and as such skin problems that have no known cause are often associated with renal dysfunction. Skin problems can also be an indication that the kidney is no longer processing metabolic waste correctly.

The kidney plays an important role in blood pressure control via the rennin-angiotensin system. Always rule out renal dysfunction with hypertension of unknown etiology. This is a very common reason for a mild to moderate elevated blood pressure, yet many patients are immediately put on medications to "normalize" blood pressure. These medications can further worsen an over-looked underlying renal insufficiency.

| **Dehydration**
 | If BUN is increased suspect dehydration. Dehydration is a very common problem and should be factored into your blood chemistry and CBC analysis. **Please see special topic on dehydration on page 90 for more details.**

Pattern:

 Suspect a short-term (acute) dehydration if there is an increased HGB (>14.5 or 145 in women or 15 or 150 in men) and/or HCT (>44 or 0.44 in women and >48 or 0.48 in men) along with an increased RBC count (>4.5 in women and >4.9 in men). A relative increase in Sodium (>142) and Potassium (>4.5) can be noted as well.

 Suspect a long-term (chronic) dehydration if any of the |

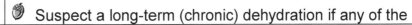

	above findings are accompanied by an increased Albumin (>5.0 or 50 g/L), increased BUN (>16 or 5.71 mmol/L) and/or serum Protein (>7.4 or 74 g/L).
Hypochlorhydria	An increased BUN level is often associated with a decreased production of hydrochloric acid in the stomach (hypochlorhydria), which leads to increased levels of undigested protein in the intestines and greatly predisposes one towards the development of a dysbiotic bowel with an overgrowth of bacteria. Putrefactive action of this bacterial overgrowth on the excess nitrogenous waste releases significant quantities of ammonia. Some of this ammonia will be converted into urea by the liver. Increased bacteria in the colon will also metabolize urea often leading to an increased BUN.
	Please see the special topic on hypochlorhydria on page 96 for more details.
	<u>Pattern</u>:
	Hypochlorhydria is **possible** with an increased globulin level (>2.8 or 28 g/L) and a normal or decreased Total Protein/Albumin.
	Hypochlorhydria is **probable** if globulin levels are increased (>2.8 or 28 g/L)along with an increased BUN (>16 or 5.71 mmol/L), a decreased or normal Total Protein/Albumin and/or decreased serum Phosphorous (<3.0 or 0.97 mmol/L).
	Other values that may be reflective of a developing or chronic hypochlorhydria include increased or decreased gastrin (<50 or >100), an increased MCV (>90) and MCH (>31.9), a decreased or normal calcium (<9.2 or 2.3 mmol/L) and iron (<50 or 8.96 μmol/dL), a decreased chloride (<100), an increased anion gap (>12) and a decreased alkaline phosphatase (<70).
	Some of clinical indications of Hypochlorhydria include:
	1. Gas and bloating shortly after meals
	2. Sense of fullness/ Easy satiety
	3. Nausea after taking supplements
	4. Weak, peeling or cracked nails
	5. Dilated capillaries in cheeks and nose in non-alcoholics
Diet- excessive protein intake or catabolism	Since the BUN level is dependent on dietary protein, an increased dietary protein or an increased catabolism of protein will lead to an increased BUN level.

Adrenal hyperfunction	BUN levels will be increased in states of protein catabolism, which is increased in adrenal hyperfunction. Excess cortisol levels will cause mobilization and an increased level of amino acids in the blood and liver by promoting protein catabolism. This will increase the levels of BUN. Adrenal hyperfunction is often due to stress, excess physical activity, blood sugar dysregulation, and chronic inflammation.
Dysbiosis	An increased BUN level can be caused by a dysbiotic bowel, due to an overgrowth of bacteria. In the large intestine, putrefactive action of this bacterial overgrowth on nitrogenous materials releases significant quantities of ammonia. Some of this ammonia will be converted into urea by the liver. A significant amount of urea also travels from the liver to the colon and is acted upon by gut microflora to recirculate nitrogen. Increased catabolism of that urea in the colonic environment will increase the BUN.
Edema	An increased BUN is associated with edema. Edema is rarely primary and is most often secondary to other metabolic disturbances, e.g. renal dysfunction, food/environmental sensitivities, cardiac muscle stress, or endocrine dysfunction. Investigate with appropriate testing (i.e. cardiac, hormone, and allergy testing). Serum sodium levels may also be decreased.
Anterior pituitary dysfunction	An increased BUN above 25 or 8.93 mmol/L should be viewed as a sign of renal dysfunction. In cases of renal dysfunction the serum creatinine will most likely be elevated. If the serum creatinine is not above 1.1 and the BUN is elevated consider that the problem may be due to an anterior pituitary dysfunction and not renal dysfunction.
Drug causes of ↑	❋ Diuretics (used for edema or hypertension) ❋ Prescription corticosteroids (i.e. Prednisone, Prednisolone) ❋ Many other drugs can lead to an elevated BUN
Other conditions associated with increased BUN levels include	Gout ❋ CHF Decreased protein utilization ❋ Gastric bleeding Boron deficiency

LOW

Clinical Implication	Additional information
Diet- low protein	A decreased BUN level is associated with a diet that is low in protein. The amount of urea excreted as BUN varies with the amount of dietary protein intake. Low protein diets may show up with a decreased BUN level (<10 or 3.57 mmol/L) and a decreased BUN/Creatinine ratio (<10).
Malabsorption	A decreased BUN (<10 or 3.57 mmol/L) is associated with a chronic intestinal malabsorption, which is an inability of nutrients to be absorbed through the intestinal wall. Malabsorption can lead to a functional protein deficit, which in turn will lead to lower levels of protein catabolism and low BUN levels.
	Malabsorption is characterized by the abnormal excretion of fat in the stool and the malabsorption of macronutrients, especially protein. Some of the causes of malabsorption include enzyme deficiency which can lead to defective protein breakdown, diarrhea, or an increased bowel transit time, and decreased surface area of the intestinal lumen, a condition associated with Celiac's disease.
Pancreatic insufficiency	A decreased BUN (<10 or 3.57 mmol/L) is associated with a pancreatic insufficiency. A decreased level of digestive enzymes secreted from the pancreas, especially protease, can lead to a functional protein deficit. This in turn will lead to lower levels of protein catabolism and low BUN levels.
	Some of the clinical implications of pancreatic insufficiency include: 1. Undigested food in the stool 2. Food allergies 3. Indigestion, gas, bloating 4. Diarrhea 5. Sense of excess fullness after meals 6. Sleepy after meals especially one high in carbohydrates
Liver dysfunction	A decreased BUN (<10 or 3.57 mmol/L) is associated with liver dysfunction. Dysfunction in the liver will have a great impact on protein production and synthesis, which will affect the availability of protein for catabolism, resulting in low BUN levels.
	Functionally oriented liver problems, such as detoxification

	issues, liver congestion, and conjugation problems are extremely common and should be evaluated based upon early prognostic indicators. The liver should always be viewed in the context of the hepato-biliary tree. Some of the key clinical indicators include: 1. Pain between shoulder blades 2. Stomach upset by greasy foods 3. If drinking alcohol, easily intoxicated 4. Headache over the eye 5. Sensitive to chemicals (perfume, cleaning solvents, insecticides, exhaust, etc.) 6. Hemorrhoids or varicose veins
Posterior pituitary dysfunction	A decreased BUN (<10 or 3.57 mmol/L) along with a decreased urinary specific gravity and a decreased BUN/Creatinine ratio that is below 10 can be an indication of dysfunction in the posterior pituitary, which is responsible for the production of Anti Diuretic Hormone (ADH).
Drug causes of ↓	✳ Anabolic steroids ✳ Some antibiotics
Other conditions associated with decreased BUN levels include	🝆 Dysbiosis 🝆 Pregnancy ✳ Anabolic steroid use ✳ Liver failure ✳ Severe liver disease

Interfering Factors:

Falsely increased levels	Falsely decreased levels
• Late pregnancy (due to increased use of protein)	• Small muscle mass (e.g. women and children)

Related Tests:

Serum creatinine, urinary uric acid, blood electrolytes, SGPT/ALT, SGOT/AST, GGTP, serum ALP, isoenzymes of ALP, MCV/MCH, RBC, HCT and ROB, sedimentation rate, basophils, gamma globulin, rheumatoid factor, serum phosphorous, CDSA, hair-mineral analysis, and urinary heavy metal screen.

Creatinine

Background

Creatinine is a by-product of muscle creatine phosphate breakdown during muscle contraction. Creatine phosphate acts as a storage depot for muscle energy. It is produced primarily from the contraction of muscle. Its production is dependent on the muscle mass of the person, and is removed by the kidneys.

Discussion

 Serum Creatinine levels are affected by the muscle mass of the individual. Patients with increased muscle mass may have slightly higher creatinine levels while patients with decreased muscle mass (older adults and children) may have lower levels.

- A disorder of the kidney and/or urinary tract will reduce the excretion of creatinine and thus raise blood serum levels. Creatinine, unlike BUN, is not affected by gender or the amount of dietary protein consumed. Conditions that cause excess protein breakdown (tissue destruction, inflammation, cancer etc.) will not cause increased creatinine levels.

- Creatinine is traditionally used with BUN to assess impaired kidney function. It is a more specific and sensitive test indicator of renal disease than BUN.

- Creatinine levels above 1.1 can be used as a prognostic indicator for potential problems in the uterus or prostate (Benign Prostatic Hypertrophy, uterine congestion, uterine hypertrophy). This is more likely if other causes for a creatinine increase have been ruled-out e.g. renal disease, prescription drugs. An increased PSA will often show a prostate condition in its later stages.

Ranges:

	Standard U.S. Units	Standard International Units
Conventional Laboratory Range	0.6 – 1.5 mg/dL	53.0 – 132.6 µmol/L
Optimal Range	0.8 - 1.1 mg/dL	70.7 – 97.2 µmol/L
Alarm Ranges	> 1.6 mg/dL	>141.4 µmol/L

When would you run this test?

1. To assess kidney function

2. To assess prostate and uterine function

3. To monitor prostate treatments

4. To monitor IV chelation treatments

Clinical implications

HIGH

Clinical Implication	Additional information
MALE **Urinary Tract Congestion or Obstruction** • **Benign Prostatic Hypertrophy (BPH)** • **Prostatitis** • **UTI**	Congestion or obstruction in the urinary tract will cause a back-up into the kidneys, impacting normal renal function. This can lead to an accumulation of creatinine in the blood and may be indicative of a chronic inflammatory, infectious or obstructive process (i.e. BPH, prostatitis, chronic UTIs). If the serum creatinine is 1.2 or higher in a male over 40 years old, prostatic hypertrophy must be considered. Often the creatinine will increase long before the PSA increases. **Pattern:** Suspect BPH if there is an increased creatinine level (>1.1 or 97.2μmol/dL) along with a normal BUN and electrolytes The likelihood of BPH increases when there is an increased creatinine level (>1.1 or 97.2μmol/dL), along with a normal BUN and electrolytes, and an increased monocyte count (>7%) and LDH isoenzyme #4, which has a prostatic origin. **If BPH is suspected the following may be indicated:** a microscopic examination of the urine for prostate cells, a urinalysis indicating infection, and a prostate exam. Some of the key clinical indications of a developing prostate problem include: 1. Difficulty urinating and/or dribbling 2. Difficulty starting and stopping urine stream 3. Waking to urinate at night 4. Interruption of stream during urination 5. Unresolved back pain and/or pain on inside of heels 6. Feeling of incomplete bowel evacuation 7. Erectile dysfunction

Renal disease	The pattern found below is indicative of an impaired renal function, which should be ruled-out or referred to a qualified practitioner if present. However, an elevated BUN found in isolation of the pattern below is more indicative of renal insufficiency or other causes. **Pattern:** Increased BUN (>25 or 8.93 mmol/L) serum creatinine (>1.4 or >123.8 μmol/dL) BUN/Creatinine ratio (10-20), Urine specific gravity (1.010 - 1.016), Uric acid (>5.9 or > 351 μmol/dL), serum phosphorous (>4.0 or 1.29 mmol/L), LDH (>200), and SGOT/AST (>30).
Renal insufficiency	A normal or increased serum Creatinine (>1.1 or 97.2μmol/dL) can be a sign of renal insufficiency. Renal insufficiency is an often over-looked condition. **Please see the special topic on page 40 for more details.** **Pattern:** Suspect renal insufficiency if there is an increased BUN level (>16 or 5.71 mmol/L) with a normal or increased serum Creatinine (>1.1 or 97.2μmol/dL), a normal to increased Uric Acid (>5.9 or > 351 μmol/dL), and an increased serum phosphorous (>4.0 or 1.29 mmol/L). LDH and SGOT/AST will usually be normal.
FEMALE **Urinary Tract Congestion or Obstruction** ● **Uterine hypertrophy** ● **Uterine inflammation** ● **UTI**	Congestion or obstruction in the urinary tract can be caused by uterine hypertrophy or inflammation, which will cause a back-up into the kidneys, impacting normal renal function. This can lead to an accumulation of creatinine in the blood and may be indicative of a chronic inflammatory, infectious or obstructive process **Pattern:** Suspect urinary tract obstruction or congestion due to uterine hypertrophy or inflammation if there is an increased creatinine level (>1.1 or 97.2μmol/dL) along with a normal BUN and electrolytes
Drug causes of ↑	❈ Aspirin/NSAIDS ❈ Indomethacin ❈ Antibiotics ❈ Diuretics (Furosamide, thiazide, etc.) ❈ Bismuth ❈ Lithium

Other conditions associated with increased serum creatinine levels include	Urinary tract obstruction	Uncontrolled diabetes
	Dehydration	Congestive heart failure
	Creatine supplementation	

LOW

Clinical Implication	Additional information
Muscle Atrophy/Nerve-Muscle Degeneration	Due to its connection to muscle metabolism serum creatinine will be decreased in cases of muscle atrophy or nerve-muscle degeneration
Other conditions associated with decreased serum creatinine levels include	Little metabolism in the muscles indicating a need for exercise · Liver disease · Muscular dystrophy · Multiple sclerosis

Interfering Factors:

Drugs that influence kidney function can cause a change in serum creatinine

Falsely increased levels	Falsely decreased levels
• High ascorbic acid intake	• High bilirubin levels
• Cephalosporin antibiotics	• Cephalosporin antibiotics
• A diet high in meat may cause increased levels	• Glucose, histidine, and quinidine compounds

Related Tests:

BUN, creatinine clearance, uric acid, blood electrolytes, Prostatic Specific Antigen (PSA), liver enzymes, urinalysis.

BUN/Creatinine Ratio

Discussion

The BUN/Creatinine is dependent on the BUN and Creatinine levels. It should be used as a rough guide, due to the variability in BUN and Creatinine levels, and should always be viewed in context with BUN and Creatinine. Use the ratio to assess patients with chronic renal dysfunction.

- An increased ratio is usually due to either a decreased Creatinine or an increased BUN level

- A decreased ratio is usually due to either a BUN decrease with a Creatinine increase or a normal BUN with a greatly increased Creatinine.

Ranges:

	Standard U.S. Units	Standard International Units
Conventional Laboratory Range	6 – 20	7 – 14
Optimal Range	10 – 16	13 – 17
Alarm Ranges	< 5 or >30	< 4 or > 31

When would you run this test?

1. This test is useful when assessing patients with chronic renal dysfunction.

Clinical implications

HIGH

Clinical Implication	Additional information
Renal disease	The pattern found below is indicative of an impaired renal function. This should be ruled out and referred to a qualified practitioner if this pattern is present. However, an elevated BUN found in isolation of the pattern below is more indicative of renal insufficiency or other causes.
	Pattern:
	Increased BUN (>25 or 8.93 mmol/L) serum creatinine (>1.4 or >123.8 µmol/dL), BUN/Creatinine ratio (10-20), Urine

	specific gravity (1.010 - 1.016), Uric acid (>5.9 or 351 μmol/dL), serum phosphorous (>4.0 or 1.29 mmol/L), LDH (>200), and SGOT/AST (>30).
Drug causes of ↓	❄ Steroids ❄ Antibiotics
Other conditions associated with ↑ BUN/Creatinine ratio include	🍂 High protein intake ❄ GI bleeding 🍂 Dehydration

LOW

Clinical Implication	Additional information
Diet- Low protein	A decreased BUN level (<10 or 3.57 mmol/L) is associated with a diet that is low in protein. The amount of urea excreted as BUN varies with the amount of dietary protein intake, therefore low protein diets may show up with a decreased BUN level and a decreased BUN/Creatinine ratio.
Posterior pituitary dysfunction	A BUN/Creatinine ratio decreased below 10 may be an indication of inappropriate secretion of anti-diuretic hormone (ADH -Vasopressin) due to posterior pituitary dysfunction. You may also see a decreased BUN (<10 or 3.57 mmol/L) along with a decreased urinary specific gravity.
Drug causes of ↓	❄ Cephalosporin (antibiotics) ❄ Phenacemide (anti-convulsant)
Other conditions associated with decreased BUN/Creatinine ratio include	🍂 Pregnancy (normal) ❄ Diabetic acidosis 🍂 Liver dysfunction ❄ Dialysis

Interfering Factors:

Falsely increased levels	Falsely decreased levels
• None noted	• None noted

Related Tests:

BUN, Creatinine, uric acid

Uric Acid

Background

Uric acid is produced as an end product of purine, nucleic acid, and nucleoprotein metabolism. Levels represent the end product of protein utilization and deamination in the liver. The kidneys store and excrete about 2/3^{rds} of the uric acid produced daily, making it an indirect marker of renal function as well. The remaining 1/3rd is excreted in the stool. Uric acid is the end-product of xanthine oxidase activation and reduced tissue oxygenation will induce its production. An over-production of uric acid occurs in conditions of excessive breakdown and catabolism of nucleic acids, increased destruction of cells and an inability to adequately excrete uric acid.

Discussion

The conventional focus of uric acid measurement is for gout, renal failure, and leukemia. However, this marker is a very strong indicator for potential inflammation and metabolic disturbance.

- When inflammation is present the body wants to start laying down protective tissue (bone spurs, atherosclerosis, fibrosis etc.) and this activates xanthine oxidase pathways causing increased uric acid levels.

- Dietary purines from dark meat, organ meats, pork, shellfish, legumes etc. may be a cause of increased uric acid levels and should therefore be limited when treating patients with elevated uric acid levels. However, chemical and physical stressors are the most common reasons for an elevation.

- There are many potential interferences for uric acid levels as it is quite labile. As a result, serial measurements are most useful for making clinical inferences. Daily and seasonal variations, obesity, stress levels etc. all can play a major role in its metabolism.

- Over ¾ of patients with heart disease and high triglycerides will present with elevated levels of uric acid. The role of oxidative stress in the process of cardiovascular disease cannot be over-emphasized. Consider oxidative stress measurements with an elevated uric acid history.

Ranges:

	Standard U.S. Units	Standard International Units
Conventional Laboratory Range	2.2 – 7.7 mg/dL	131 – 458 µmol/L
Optimal Range	**Males:** 3.5 – 5.9 mg/dL **Females:** 3.0 – 5.5 mg/dL	**Males:** 208 – 351 µmol/L **Females:** 178 – 327 µmol/L
Alarm Ranges	< 2.0 or > 9.0 mg/dL	< 119 or > 535 µmol/L

When would you run this test?

1. To assist in the diagnosis of an inflammatory or circulatory disorder
2. To screen for potential developing signs of heart disease
3. As a marker for oxidative stress activity

Clinical implications

HIGH

Clinical Implication	Additional information
Gout 	Increased uric acid levels are associated with Gout, which is a condition in which uric acid crystals precipitate in the tissue, especially the big toe (tophi). **Pattern:** If there is an increased uric acid (>5.9 or > 351 µmol/dL), Gout is **possible**. The likelihood increases if there is also a decreased phosphorous (<3.0 or <0.97 mmol/L), an increased cholesterol (>220 or 5.69 mmol/L), BUN (>16 or 5.71 mmol/L) and a normal or increased creatinine (>1.1 or 97.2µmol/dL). **Please see the special topic below for more information.**

> # "Sub-Acute Gout"
>
> Many arthralgias are actually a form of "sub-acute gout". Patients who are unresponsive to treatment for an assumed arthritis, fibromyalgia, or any migrating

joint pain or stiffness/inflammation should be considered for this metabolic problem. "Sub-acute gout" is actually quite common. A patient may in fact be suffering from a "sub-acute gout" even when the uric acid is not elevated above the reference range and the big toe is not swollen.

A low purine diet is critical in addition to the elimination of refined carbohydrates, alcohol, fried, processed or hydrogenated foods, and caffeine. Water intake should be emphasized.

Treatment considerations should include B-complex, Folic acid (prevents crystal formation), organic Lithium (breaks down crystals), and magnesium.

Atherosclerosis	An increased uric acid level is associated with chronic inflammatory states including those in the vascular system. This is one of the precipitating factors in the development of atherosclerosis. Over ¾ of patients with heart disease and high triglycerides will present with elevated levels of uric acid. Oxidative stress plays a large role in the process of cardiovascular disease. Please see the section below on uric acid and oxidative stress. Atherosclerosis is particularly accelerated in individuals with increased oxidative stress, a clinical presentation of metabolic syndrome, B-vitamin metabolism problems, and familial hyperlipidemia. **Pattern:** If there is an increased uric acid level (>5.9 or > 351 μmol/dL) with an increased triglyceride (>200 or 2.26 mmol/L) in relation to total cholesterol (>220 or 5.69 mmol/L), a decreased HDL (<45 or 1.16 mmol/L) and an increased LDL (>120 or 3.1 mmol/L), atherosclerosis is **probable**. Platelet levels may also be increased (>385). Homocysteine levels are frequently increased with atherosclerosis. If the above pattern is not present and the uric acid level is elevated (>5.9 or > 351 μmol/dL) still consider running a serum homocysteine, as a homocysteinuria may be the locus of a developing problem.
Oxidative Stress and Free Radical Activity	Suspect excess free radical activity and oxidative stress if the Uric acid level is elevated. **Pattern:** If the uric acid level is increased (>5.9 or > 351 μmol/dL) with a total cholesterol level that is suddenly below its historical level, a decreased lymphocyte count (<20), a decreased

	albumin (<4.0 or 40g/L) and platelet level (<150), and an increased total globulin (>2.8 or 28 g/L) free radical pathology, which increases the risk for developing a neoplasm, should be investigated. This can be accomplished in the office using the Oxidata free radical test. **Please see page 152 for a discussion of this test.** Oxidative stress can cause an increased destruction of red blood cells; in these situations you will see an elevated bilirubin level (>1.2 or 20.5µmol/dL).
Rheumatoid Arthritis 	Increased uric acid levels are associated with chronic inflammation and commonly present in conditions such as Rheumatoid Arthritis. The following are contributing factors for the development of Rheumatoid Arthritis and should be investigated and treated appropriately: 1. Viral, yeast, and bacterial infection 2. Chronic hypochlorhydria 3. Intestinal and systemic parasites (consider amoebic origin) 4. Intestinal dysbiosis 5. Food and environmental sensitivity 6. Heavy metals If there are clinical indications of joint pain and/or inflammation and you see the following pattern consider that there may be a developing Rheumatoid Arthritis: **Pattern:** A developing rheumatoid arthritis may be seen with an increased uric acid level (>5.9 or > 351 µmol/dL), an increased ESR, a decreased or normal albumin (<4.0 or 40g/L), alkaline phosphatase (<70) and increased or normal serum calcium (>10.0 or 2.5 mmol/L). Consider following up with any one of the following tests or with a Rheumatoid panel to help delineate the nature of the arthralgias. C-Complement increased when active, decreased when in remission, C-reactive protein increased, Rheumatoid factor normal or increased, Alpha-2 increased in acute phase, Gamma Globulin increased in chronic phase), Homocysteine increased. A normal Rheumatoid factor will not necessarily rule out RA, as it is usually only elevated in more severe cases

Renal insufficiency	An increased Uric acid level can be a sign of renal insufficiency. Renal insufficiency is an often over-looked condition. **Please see the special topic on page 40 for more details.** **Pattern:** Suspect renal insufficiency if there is an increased BUN level (>16 or 5.71 mmol/L) with a normal or increased serum creatinine (>1.1 or 97.2μmol/dL), a normal to increased uric acid (>5.9 or 351 μmol/dL), and an increased serum phosphorous (>4.0 or 1.29 mmol/L). LDH and SGOT/AST will usually be normal.
Renal disease	Increased uric acid levels are associated with decreased renal function. The pattern found below is indicative of an impaired renal function, which should be ruled-out or referred to a qualified practitioner if present. **Pattern:** Increased BUN (>25 or 8.93 mmol/L) serum creatinine (>1.4 or >123.8 μmol/dL) BUN/creatinine ratio (10-20), urine specific gravity (1.010 - 1.016 Uric acid (>5.9 or 351 μmol/dL), serum phosphorous (>4.0 or 1.29 mmol/L), LDH (>200), and SGOT/AST (>30).
Circulatory disorders	Patients with increased uric acid levels should be evaluated for circulatory disorders. The enzyme Xanthine oxidase, which is essential for the formation of uric acid, is activated with poor circulation producing elevated uric acid levels as well as a super oxide radical. Conditions such as **Hypertension**, **Raynaud's**, **Atherosclerosis**, and **Polycythemia** should be considered and treated appropriately.
"Leaky Gut" syndrome	Consider an altered intestinal permeability when the uric acid levels are high (>5.9 or 351 μmol/dL) and an underlying inflammatory problem is present. Many organisms (bacteria, yeast, amoebas) and their toxins are easily absorbed in a compromised digestive barrier, setting up a resultant auto-immune response in many cases. Treatment should be oriented to restoring gut integrity and correcting the dysbiotic terrain. Note that a reaction is common initially (Herxheimer reaction) as an increased release of endotoxins occurs during early treatment.
Drug and toxicity causes of ↑	✳ Drug diuretics (especially thiazides)

	❋ Aspirin (even low dose)
	❋ Theophylline, caffeine, theobromine (coffee, tea, colas)
	❋ Heavy metal body burden (or decreased)
Other conditions associated with increased uric acid levels include	🖐 Para-thyroid hyperfunction ❋ Diabetes 🖐 Liver/Biliary dysfunction ❋ Congestive heart failure 🖐 Thyroid hypofunction ❋ Neoplasm 🖐 "Stress" – treat with appropriate lifestyle and diet modifications ❋ Polycythemia ❋ Inflammatory conditions (arthralgias etc…) 🖐 ↑ Dietary purines (pork, organ meats, shellfish, legumes, sweetbreads etc.) ❋ Acidosis ❋ Fasting ❋ Lead poisoning

LOW

Clinical Implication	Additional information
Molybdenum Deficiency	Xanthine oxidase contains molybdenum and is the enzyme that converts purine bases into Uric acid. It has a wide distribution in the body, occurring in breast milk, small intestine, kidneys and the liver, where it is integral to phase II liver detoxification pathways. A very common deficiency in this mineral will compromise Xanthine oxidase activity leading to a decreased Uric acid. **Pattern**: Suspect molybdenum deficiency if there is a decreased uric acid level (<3.5 or 208 mmol/L) and a normal MCV and MCH Rule out Molybdenum deficiency if the following indications are present: ● Sensitivity to exhaust fumes and gases ● Sensitivity to perfumes and fragrances ● Sensitive to MSG, sulfites used in food preparation (red wines, hot dogs etc.)

Anemia- B12/Folate Deficiency 	A decreased uric acid level is associated with a chronic B12/folate anemia. By no means a sole diagnostic indicator, it should be viewed in context with the appropriate red blood cell indices (RBCs, MCV, MCH, and MCHC) and a methylmelonic acid test. B12/Folate deficiency may be due to a number of different factors: • **Decreased ingestion:** vegan diet • **Impaired absorption:** Intrinsic factor deficiency, pernicious anemia, malabsorption, HCl need, hypochlorhydria • **Competitive parasites** • **Increased requirements:** Chronic pancreatic disease, pregnancy, hyperthyroidism • **Impaired utilization:** enzyme deficiencies, abnormal binding proteins
Copper Deficiency 	Low Uric acid levels have been associated with a potential copper deficiency. Copper is required for the formation of hemoglobin, adrenal hormones, bone matrix, several enzymes of detoxification formed in the liver, and the formation of high density lipoproteins (HDL). A chronic iron deficiency anemia may actually indicate a copper problem as copper is required for proper iron uptake and utilization. Poor skin and connective tissue integrity as well as chronic adrenal problems may result from a long-standing copper deficit as well. Clinical indications of a potential copper deficiency include: 1. Fatigue and energy problems 2. Chronic anemia (iron) 3. Easy bruising (ruptured blood vessels) 4. Osteoporosis or poor bone density 5. Bone and Joint abnormalities 6. Impaired immune function **However, copper is an extremely toxic element when found in excess. Do not supplement without reasonable cause.** Confirm levels with a WBC intracellular level as serum and hair mineral testing are not reliable for this element.

Pregnancy	Uric acid is valuable in assessing the prognosis of eclampsia because of the uric acid levels ability to reflect the extent of liver damage in toxemia of pregnancy. **Please see the special topic on Pregnancy and its impact on Laboratory Values on page 94 for more details.**
Drug and toxicity causes of ↓	❋ Aspirin (high doses) ❋ Corticosteroids ❋ Heavy metal poisoning
Other conditions associated with decreased uric acid levels include	Wilson's disease ❋ Obstructive Liver Disease Familial periodic paralysis ❋ Neoplasm Improper RBC production ❋ Fanconi's syndrome

Interfering Factors:

Falsely increased levels	Falsely decreased levels
• Stress and strenuous exercise will elevate a uric acid level	• None noted

Related Tests:

Serum creatinine, BUN, Blood electrolytes, ALT, AST, GGTP, serum ALP, ALP isoenzymes, MCV, MCH, RBC, HCT, HGB, ESR, Basophils, gamma Globulin, Rheumatoid factor, Phosphorous, heavy metal screening, Homocysteine, C reactive protein

Potassium

Background

Potassium is the main intracellular cation, and acts as the primary intracellular pH buffer. The majority of potassium (90%) is found inside the cell, with only small amounts found in other tissues, such as bone and blood. Intracellular potassium concentration can be as much as 15 to 20 times greater than the serum/plasma. Due to the critical functions of potassium for human metabolism and physiology it is essential for the body to maintain optimum serum levels even though a small concentration is found outside of the cell.

Potassium plays an essential role in nerve conduction, the maintenance of osmotic pressure, muscle function, cellular transport via the sodium-potassium pump, and acid-base balance. Potassium, along with calcium and magnesium, controls the rate and force of cardiac muscle contraction and thus controls cardiac output.

Potassium, along with sodium, plays an important role in the kidney's regulation of pH. Potassium bicarbonate is the major intracellular inorganic buffer. When the body is deficient in potassium, intracellular acidosis occurs. The body responds by acting on the respiratory center to increase the respiration rate and depth of breathing. This increases carbon dioxide excretion and brings the body back into pH balance.

Potassium excretion is controlled primarily by the kidney. Between 80 – 90% of cellular potassium is excreted from the kidney in the urine, the remainder is excreted in the sweat and stool. The kidney does not conserve potassium and will continue to excrete potassium, even when an adequate amount of potassium is not consumed. Thus, a potassium deficiency can occur if adequate amounts of potassium are not consumed on a daily basis.

Discussion

 As the chief cation found in the intracellular fluid, potassium levels will increase with cellular damage, which causes the potassium to leach into the extracellular fluid.

- Potassium concentration is greatly influenced by adrenal hormones, especially aldosterone. Aldosterone causes an increased excretion of potassium from the urine. As such, potassium levels can be a marker for adrenal dysfunction.

- Potassium levels should always be viewed in relation to the other electrolytes

Common subjective indications of potassium need are:

1. Muscle weakness
2. Fatigue
3. Mental confusion
4. Heart disturbances
5. Problems in nerve conduction.

Ranges:

	Standard U.S. Units	**Standard International Units**
Conventional Laboratory Range	3.5 – 5.3 mEq/L	3.5 – 5.3 mmol/L
Optimal Range	4.0 – 4.5 mEq/L	4.0 – 4.5 mmol/L
Alarm Ranges	< 3.0 or > 6.0 mEq/L	< 3.0 or > 6.0 mmol/L

When would you run this test?

1. As a marker for adrenal health

2. Acid-base balance

Clinical implications

HIGH

Clinical Implication	**Additional information**
Adrenal Hypofunction	Adrenal hypofunction can cause a decrease in the secretions of both the glucocorticoid and mineralcorticoid hormones. A decrease in aldosterone, the major mineralcorticoid, from adrenal hypofunction will have an impact on potassium metabolism. Decreased aldosterone levels will cause a decrease in the amount of renal potassium excretion, which will cause an increase in serum potassium. **Pattern:** If the potassium levels (>4.5) are increased along with a normal or decreased sodium (< 135) and/or chloride (<100), adrenal hypofunction is **possible**. Other values that may be out of balance include decreased aldosterone and cortisol levels. Urinary chloride will be increased.

61

	Adrenal hypofunction can be confirmed with salivary cortisol studies. Some of the clinical signs of adrenal hypofunction include: 1. Low systolic blood pressure 2. Craving for salt 3. Chronic fatigue 4. Afternoon yawning 5. Weakness and dizziness 6. Extreme fatigue after exercise 7. Poor circulation 8. Weakness after colds or flu, slow to recover
Dehydration	If potassium is increased (>4.5) suspect dehydration. Dehydration is a very common problem and should be factored into your blood chemistry and CBC analysis. **Please see special topic on page 90 for more details.** **Pattern:** Suspect a short-term (acute) dehydration if there is an increased HGB (>14.5 or 145 in women or 15 or 150 in men) and/or HCT (>44 or 0.44 in women and >48 or 0.48 in men) along with an increased RBC count (>4.5 in women and >4.9 in men). A relative increase in sodium (>142) and potassium (>4.5) can be noted as well. Suspect a long-term (chronic) dehydration if any of the above findings are accompanied by an increased albumin (>4.8 or 48 g/L), BUN (>16 or 5.71 mmol/L), and/or serum protein (>7.4 or 74 g/L).
Tissue destruction	Potassium is an intracellular ion. An increase in tissue destruction can cause an increase in serum potassium levels as the potassium is leached out of the damaged cells. LDH (> 200) levels may also be elevated. Follow-up suspected tissue destruction with serum protein and LDH isoenzyme electrophoresis, which can help pin point the specific tissue that is being affected.
Metabolic Acidosis	Metabolic acidosis will drive potassium out of the cell, thus causing an increase in serum potassium.
Other conditions associated with increased levels include	Respiratory distress Bradycardia Renal failure Diabetes Renal insufficiency Addison's disease

LOW

Clinical Implication	Additional information
Adrenal Hyperfunction	Adrenal hyperfunction can cause an increase in the secretions of both the glucocorticoid and mineralcorticoid hormones. An increase in aldosterone, the major mineralcorticoid, from adrenal hyperfunction will have an impact on potassium metabolism. Increased aldosterone levels will cause an increase in the amount of renal potassium excretion, which will cause a decrease in serum potassium. **Pattern:** If the potassium levels are decreased (<4.0) along with a normal or increased sodium (>142), and/or chloride (>106), adrenal hyperfunction is **possible**. Other values that may be out of balance include increased aldosterone and cortisol levels. If the cortisol level is significantly elevated, rule out adrenal adenoma. Urinary chloride will be decreased. Adrenal hyperfunction can be confirmed with salivary cortisol studies. Some of the clinical signs of adrenal hyperfunction include: 1. High blood pressure 2. Headaches 3. Hot flashes 4. Excessive hair growth on face or body (females) 5. Keyed up, trouble calming down 6. Clench or grind teeth
Drug Diuretics	Many of the diuretic drugs are potassium sparing. Even so, serum potassium can be decreased with the use of these drugs. In these cases the BUN (>16 or 5.71 mmol/L) and creatinine (>1.1 or 97.2µmol/dL) will frequently be increased, indicating renal insufficiency, and sodium will be decreased. On the other hand, it is important to not presume that a patient needs potassium because they are on a drug diuretic. Prolonged diuretic use may also deplete thiamine.
Benign Essential Hypertension	Benign Essential Hypertension is common with decreased potassium, even when cortisol, renin and other indicators may be normal. Generally, increased potassium suggests a congestive heart problem, and decreased potassium suggests a fatigued heart muscle. HTN has many potential causes and should be investigated with other methodologies beyond blood chemistries.

Other conditions associated with decreased potassium levels include	Anemia (many types) Diets high in refined CHOs Excessive licorice consumption (herbal)	Acute and chronic diarrhea Hypertension Familial periodic paralysis

Interfering Factors:

Falsely increased levels	Falsely decreased levels
• Hemolyzed blood – potassium levels are elevated up to 50% of normal with even moderate hemolysis. Making a fist ten times with a tourniquet in place alone may result in an increased level of 10-20% • Excessive intake of licorice (herbal)	• Glucose administered during tolerance testing, or the ingestion and administration of large amounts of glucose in patients with heart disease may decrease levels by up to 0.4 mmol/L

Related Tests:

Plasma and salivary cortisol, blood aldosterone, plasma rerun, serum calcium, serum chloride, serum sodium, CO_2 and anion gap; HGB, HCT and RBC, serum BUN, serum creatinine, serum and salivary dehydroepiandrosterone (DHEA).

Sodium

Background

Constituting 90% of the electrolyte fluid, sodium is the most prevalent cation in the extra-cellular fluid. Sodium acts as the chief base of the blood and functions to maintain osmotic pressure, acid-base balance, aids in nerve impulse transmission, as well as renal, cardiac and adrenal functions.

Sodium is a major part of the sodium-potassium pump, which facilitates cellular transport. Sodium also maintains the acidity of the urine.

The body has many complex mechanisms for maintaining a constant and steady level of plasma and extracellular sodium. These complex mechanisms include:

- Renal blood flow
- Carbonic anhydrase enzymatic activity
- Aldosterone
- Renin enzymatic secretion
- Antidiuretic hormone (ADH)/ Vasopressin

Discussion

Serum sodium levels are affected more by changes in fluid balance, body water and functional issues, such as adrenal dysfunction than by changes in sodium/salt balance. Urinary sodium is a more sensitive indicator of altered sodium/salt balance than blood.

- Sodium levels are ultimately under the influence of adrenal cortex hormones, especially the mineralcorticoid aldosterone, which allows the body to hold onto sodium by causing a decreased excretion of sodium from the urine. As such, sodium levels can be a marker for adrenal dysfunction.

- Increased sodium is uncommon and is most often due dehydration (sweating, diarrhea, vomiting, polyuria, etc.)

When would you run this test?

1. As a marker for adrenal health
2. Acid-base balance

Ranges:

	Standard U.S. Units	Standard International Units
Conventional Laboratory Range	135 – 145 mEq/L	135 – 145 mmol/L
Optimal Range	135 – 142 mEq/L	135 – 142 mmol/L
Alarm Ranges	< 125 or > 155 mEq/L	< 125 or > 155 mmol/L

Clinical implications

HIGH

Clinical Implication	Additional information
Adrenal Hyperfunction	Adrenal hyperfunction can cause an increase in the secretions of both the glucocorticoid and mineralcorticoid hormones. An increase in aldosterone, the major mineralcorticoid, from adrenal hyperfunction will have an impact on sodium metabolism. Increased aldosterone levels will cause an increase in sodium resorption from the kidney, which will cause an increase in serum sodium. **Pattern:** If the sodium levels are increased (>142) along with a decreased potassium (<4.0), adrenal hyperfunction is **possible**. Other values that may be out of balance include increased chloride (>106), increased aldosterone and cortisol levels. If the cortisol level is significantly elevated, rule out adrenal adenoma. Urinary chloride will be decreased. Adrenal hyperfunction can be confirmed with salivary cortisol studies. Some of the clinical signs of adrenal hyperfunction include: 1. High blood pressure 2. Headaches 3. Hot flashes 4. Excessive hair growth on face or body (females) 5. Keyed up, trouble calming down 6. Clench or grind teeth

Cushing's disease	In its pathological state, severe hyperadrenia from Cushing's disease will cause increased sodium reabsorption from the kidney and decreased sodium excretion. This is in part due to the excess of both glucocorticoids and mineralcorticoids, especially aldosterone.
Dehydration	If sodium is increased suspect dehydration. Dehydration is a very common problem and should be factored into your blood chemistry and CBC analysis. **Please see special topic on page 90 for more details.** **Pattern:** Suspect a short-term (acute) dehydration if there is an increased HGB (>14.5 or 145 in women or 15 or 150 in men) and/or HCT (>44 or 0.44 in women and >48 or 0.48 in men) along with an increased RBC count (>4.5 in women and >4.9 in men). A relative increase in Sodium (>142) and Potassium (>4.5) can be noted as well. Suspect a long-term (chronic) dehydration if any of the above findings are accompanied by an increased Albumin (>5.0 or 50 g/L), increased BUN (>16 or 5.71 mmol/L) and/or serum Protein (>7.4 or 74 g/L).
Drug Causes of ↑	Steroids Aspirin NSAIDs Anti-hypertensives Laxatives
Other conditions associated with increased sodium levels include	Water softeners, high salt intake Licorice, calcium, fluorides, and iron Renal insufficiency Diabetes insipidus Primary aldosteronism

LOW

Clinical Implication	Additional information
Adrenal Hypofunction	Adrenal hypofunction can cause a decrease in the secretions of both the glucocorticoid and mineralcorticoid hormones. A decrease in aldosterone, the major mineralcorticoid, from adrenal hypofunction will have an impact on sodium metabolism. Decreased aldosterone levels will cause an increase in the amount of renal sodium excretion, which will cause a decrease in serum sodium.
	Pattern:
	If the sodium levels are decreased (<135) along with increased potassium (>4.5), adrenal hypofunction is **possible**. Other values that may be out of balance include a decreased chloride (<100), aldosterone and cortisol levels. Urinary chloride will be increased.
	Adrenal hypofunction can be confirmed with salivary cortisol studies.
	Some of the clinical signs of adrenal hypofunction include: 1. Low systolic blood pressure 2. Craving for salt 3. Chronic fatigue 4. Weakness and dizziness 5. Extreme fatigue after exercise 6. Poor circulation 7. Weakness after colds or flu, slow to recover
Addison's disease	In its pathological state, severe hypoadrenia from Addison's disease impairs sodium reabsorption and causes excess sodium excretion due to a lack of both glucocorticoids and mineralcorticoids, especially aldosterone.
Edema	Hyponatremia (a decreased sodium level) is often reflective of a relative excess of body water rather than a low total body sodium. The following are some of the conditions implicated by this pattern: • Congestive heart failure • Hypothyroidism • Nephritis/ Kidney disease
Drug Diuretics	Drug diuretics can alter sodium as well as potassium levels in the body. Many of the diuretic drugs are potassium sparing.

	Even so, serum potassium can be decreased with the use of these drugs. In these cases the BUN and creatinine will frequently be increased, indicating renal insufficiency, and sodium will be decreased. On the other hand, it is important to not presume that a patient needs potassium need because they are on a drug diuretic. Prolonged diuretic use may also deplete Thiamine.	
Drug causes of ↓ sodium	❇ Heparin ❇ Laxatives	❇ Sulfates ❇ Diuretics
Other conditions associated with decreased sodium levels include	🌰 Low salt intake (use Celtic or sea salt instead of table salt) 🌰 Pyloric spasm/ obstruction 🌰 Diarrhea & vomiting	🌰 Excess perspiration 🌰 Diabetes 🌰 Renal dysfunction 🌰 CHF

Electrolyte Formula

A relative electrolyte balance can be determined from sodium, chloride and CO_2 levels. The sum of chloride and CO_2 is subtracted from the sodium value. Although similar to the anion gap, this formula can be helpful in assessing the electrolyte balance in your patients. A good electrolyte balance exists if the the value is between 9 – 18.

$$(Na^+) - (Cl^- + CO_2) = 9 \text{ to } 18 \text{ optimally}$$

Interfering Factors:

Falsely increased levels	Falsely decreased levels
• None noted	• High triglycerides or low protein levels can cause artificially low sodium values

Related Tests:

BUN, Creatinine, serum Potassium, Chloride, CO_2, anion gap, uric acid, salivary and plasma cortisol

Chloride

Background

Chloride is the principle extracellular anion, existing in extracellular spaces in the form of sodium chloride or hydrochloric acid. Chloride is under the same influence as sodium and is affected by many of the same conditions that affect serum sodium levels, due to their reciprocal relationship. Aldosterone, which will cause an increased reabsorption of sodium from the kidney, will also cause an increase in chloride reabsorption. Chloride levels will most often change in the same direction as sodium, i.e. if the serum sodium is decreased, we can expect to see a decreased chloride level.

On the other hand chloride has an inverse relationship with CO_2 levels. Metabolic acidosis will have an increased chloride level and a decreased CO_2 level. Metabolic alkalosis will have a decreased chloride and an increased CO_2.

Discussion

Chloride helps maintain cellular integrity by playing a role in influencing osmotic pressure and acid-base balance.

- Chloride ions are excreted along with other cations, such as sodium and potassium during diuresis and are lost from the stomach during bouts of vomiting and/or diarrhea.

Ranges:

	Standard U.S. Units	Standard International Units
Conventional Laboratory Range	97 – 107 mEq/L	97 – 107 mmol/L
Optimal Range	100 – 106 mEq/L	100 – 106 mmol/L
Alarm Ranges	<90 or >115 mEq/L	<90 or >115 mmol/L

When would you run this test?

1. As a marker for hypochlorhydria
2. As a general measure of tissue acidity and alkalinity

Clinical implications

HIGH

Clinical Implication	Additional information
Metabolic Acidosis	Increased chloride levels are associated with metabolic acidosis. Chloride tends to have an inverse relationship to CO_2 levels. In metabolic acidosis CO_2 levels are decreased, therefore you might expect to see an increase in chloride. **Please see the special topic on metabolic acidosis on page 78 for more details.** **Pattern:** Metabolic acidosis is **probable** if the CO_2 is decreased (<25), along with an increased chloride (>106) and/or an increased anion gap (>12).
Adrenal Hyperfunction	Adrenal hyperfunction can cause an increase in the secretions of both the glucocorticoid and mineralcorticoid hormones. An increase in aldosterone, the major mineralcorticoid, from adrenal hyperfunction will have an impact on sodium metabolism. When aldosterone causes an increase in the reabsorption of sodium, there is an indirect effect of increasing chloride reabsorption, causing the serum chloride levels to increase. **Pattern:** If the chloride levels (>106) are increased along with increased sodium (>142) and decreased potassium (<4.0), adrenal hyperfunction is **possible**. Other values that may be increased are aldosterone and cortisol. If the cortisol level is significantly elevated, rule-out adrenal adenoma. Urinary chloride will be decreased. Adrenal hyperfunction can be confirmed with salivary cortisol studies. Some of the clinical signs of adrenal hyperfunction include: 1. High blood pressure 2. Headaches 3. Hot flashes 4. Excessive hair growth on face or body (females) 5. Keyed up, trouble calming down 6. Clench or grind teeth

Other conditions associated with increased levels include	🍁 Salicylate (aspirin) excess 🍁 Excess salt intake 🍁 Adrenal Hyperfunction 🍁 Dehydration 🍁 Parathyroid Hyperfunction	❄ Cushing's syndrome ❄ Hyperventilation (respiratory alkalosis) ❄ Diabetes insipidus ❄ Renal tubular acidosis

LOW

Clinical Implication	Additional information
Hypochlorhydria	A decreased chloride level (<100) is associated with hypochlorhydria. Chloride is one of the main elements necessary for the production of hydrochloric acid by the parietal cells of the stomach. **Pattern:** 🍁 Hypochlorhydria is **possible** with a low serum iron and an increased (> 2.8 or 28 g/L) or decreased (<2.4 or 24 g/L) total globulin. 🍁 Hypochlorhydria is **probable** if there is also an increased BUN (>16 or 5.71 mmol/L)and/or decrease in serum phosphorous (<3.0 or <0.97 mmol/L). **Please see the special topic on Hypochlorhydria on page 96 for more details.**
Metabolic Alkalosis	Decreased chloride levels are associated with metabolic alkalosis. Chloride tends to have an inverse relationship to CO_2 levels. In metabolic alkalosis CO_2 levels are increased, therefore you might expect to see a decrease in chloride. **Please see the special topic on metabolic alkalosis on page 77 for more details.** **Pattern:** 🍁 If the CO_2 is increased (>30), along with a decreased chloride (<100), metabolic alkalosis is **possible**. 🍁 If the CO_2 is increased (>30), along with a decreased chloride (<100), calcium (<9.2 or 2.3 mmol/L), and serum potassium (<4.0), metabolic alkalosis is **probable**
Adrenal Hypofunction	Adrenal hypofunction can cause a decrease in the secretions of both the glucocorticoid and mineralcorticoid hormones. A decrease in aldosterone, the major mineralcorticoid, from

	adrenal hypofunction will have an impact on sodium metabolism. When aldosterone causes an increase in the reabsorption of sodium, there is an indirect effect of increasing chloride reabsorption. The serum chloride levels will then increase.
	When decreased aldosterone levels cause an increase in the amount of renal sodium excretion, there is an indirect effect of increasing chloride excretion, which will cause a decrease in serum chloride.
	Pattern:
	If the chloride levels are decreased (<100) along with a decreased sodium (<135) and an increased potassium (>4.5), adrenal hypofunction is **possible**.
	Other values that may be out of balance include aldosterone and cortisol levels. Urinary chloride will be increased.
	Adrenal hypofunction can be confirmed with salivary cortisol studies.
	Some of the clinical signs of adrenal hypofunction include: 1. Low systolic blood pressure 2. Craving for salt 3. Chronic fatigue 4. Afternoon yawning 5. Weakness and dizziness 6. Extreme fatigue after exercise 7. Poor circulation 8. Weakness after colds or flu, slow to recover
Drug causes of ↓	Steroids Laxatives and diuretics Theophylline Bicarbonate
Other conditions associated with decreased chloride levels include	Pyloric spasm or obstruction · Respiratory distress COPD / CHF Over-hydration · Diabetes Renal dysfunction · Addison's disease Constipation · Prolonged vomiting

Interfering Factors:

Falsely increased levels	Falsely decreased levels
<ul><li>Plasma chloride levels are normally higher in infants</li><li>Short term increases seen after saline IV infusions</li></ul>	<ul><li>None noted</li></ul>

Related Tests:

Anion gap, serum CO_2, serum potassium and sodium, BUN, serum creatinine

Carbon Dioxide

Background

Carbon Dioxide, as measured on a standard chemistry panel, is really a measure of bicarbonate in the blood. The majority of CO_2 (about 75%), produced from cellular respiration, is carried in the blood as the bicarbonate ion. 5% remains in solution as dissolved CO_2 and the remaining 20% remains combined with hemoglobin and other plasma proteins. Dissolved CO_2, formed in the lungs, contributes little to the CO_2 value.

Bicarbonate is formed by the following equation:

CO_2	+	H_2O	$\Leftrightarrow$	H_2CO_3	$\Leftrightarrow$	HCO_3^-	+	H^+
Carbon Dioxide		Water		Carbonic acid		Bicarbonate ion		Hydrogen ion

Acid-Base confusion

One of the difficulties in understanding acid-base balance is confusion in the terminology, especially the term CO_2. Ideally we should refer to CO_2 in terms of CO_2 content and CO_2 gas.

1. CO_2 content refers to bicarbonate, which is an alkaline or base molecule. It is a solution and is regulated primarily by the kidneys. This is the CO_2 referred to on blood chemistry panels.

2. CO_2 gas refers to the dissolved CO_2 and is mainly acid. It is regulated by the lungs.

Both have a powerful impact on acid-base regulation and are regulated by different organ systems.

Discussion

CO_2, as bicarbonate, is available for acid-base balancing. Bicarbonate neutralizes metabolic acids, such as hydrochloric and lactic acid.

- Bicarbonate acts as one of the reserve alkaline elements in the blood. CO_2 is not a sensitive measurement of pH or carbon dioxide gas. Conditions such as respiratory and/or metabolic acidosis or alkalosis, which are conditions of primary CO_2 increase or decrease are best evaluated and followed-up with other readings and studies (i.e. serum chloride, anion gap, blood gases).

Ranges:

	Standard U.S. Units	Standard International Units
Conventional Laboratory Range	23 – 32 mEq/L	23 – 32 mmol/L
Optimal Range	25 – 30 mEq/L	25 – 30 mmol/L
Alarm Ranges	<18 or >38 mEq/L	<18 or >38 mmol/L

When would you run this test?

1. As a general measure of tissue acidity or alkalinity

Clinical implications

HIGH

Clinical Implication	Additional information
Metabolic Alkalosis	CO_2, or bicarbonate, will be increased in metabolic alkalosis. There is a steady excess of bicarbonate in relation to H+, which causes an increase in CO_2 levels. **Please see the special topic on metabolic alkalosis below for more details.** **Pattern:** ⚇ If the CO_2 is increased (>30), along with a decreased chloride (<100), metabolic alkalosis is **possible**. ⚇ If the CO_2 is increased (>30), along with a decreased chloride (<100), calcium (<9.2 or 2.3 mmol/L), and serum potassium (<4.0), metabolic alkalosis is **probable.**

Metabolic Alkalosis

In a metabolic alkalosis, there are increasing levels of bicarbonate ion in relation to H+. There are three main causes of bicarbonate increase:

1. **Direct administration or production of alkaline**- Sodium bicarbonate, or other antacids, can lead to a metabolic alkalosis. Excess bicarbonate is absorbed and the CO_2 levels begin to rise.

2. **Acid-losing alkalosis-** The loss of H+ from the stomach from chronic vomiting or pyloric stenosis is a major cause of acid-losing alkalosis. As the HCl is being lost through vomiting, the body is losing H+ but the bicarbonate remains. The CO_2 content becomes increased as the body begins to synthesize more HCL replace the H+ and the bicarbonate produced in this process begins to rise.

3. **Potassium deficient alkalosis** – This is most often caused by an excessive loss of potassium from the kidney (i.e. diuretic use or deficiency.) Intracellular potassium will move out of the cells to replace the potassium being lost in the plasma and urine. Sodium and H^+ move into the cell to replace the potassium that has moved out. This leaves a deficit of H^+ in the plasma. Also, H^+ is excreted from the kidney along with the potassium. The net result of renal and extracellular H^+ loss is an increased production of H^+ to replace that which has been lost. This results in a concomitant rise in bicarbonate or CO_2 levels.

Adrenal hyperfunction	Adrenal hyperfunction can lead to excess secretion of aldosterone. Excess aldosterone causes a large amount of sodium to be re-absorbed from the kidney tubules. The kidney begins to lose potassium and H^+ in reaction to the sodium re-absorption. The increased loss of H^+ leads to an increased production of H^+, which in turn will lead to a concomitant rise in bicarbonate (CO_2) levels.
Hypochlorhydria	Stomach HCl is produced by the conversion of H_2CO_3 into HCO_3^- and H+, catalyzed by carbonic anhydrase. The bicarbonate is kept in the blood stream and the H+ is concentrated in the parietal cells of the stomach. Hypochlorhydria is a functional decrease in H^+ in the stomach. When HCL levels are decreased the body will attempt to increase H^+ production, leading to a concomitant rise in bicarbonate in the blood. CO_2 levels will be elevated (>30). The chloride levels are often decreased in hypochlorhydria (<100).

Respiratory acidosis	The CO_2 levels are often increased in respiratory acidosis (>30), which is due to conditions that cause pulmonary retention of CO_2. Some of the conditions include asthma, high blood pressure, damage to the respiratory centers, chest trauma or paralysis (polio), chronic respiratory diseases (emphysema and pneumonia) and obstruction of the respiratory passage. The body responds by forming bicarbonate from the excess retained CO_2 and by excreting H^+.	
Other conditions associated with increased levels include	🌰 Fever 🌰 Hot baths 🌰 Vomiting (loss of HCL)	⚕ Emphysema (Respiratory distress) ⚕ Aldosteronism ⚕ Diuretics

LOW

Clinical Implication	Additional information
Metabolic Acidosis 	CO_2, or bicarbonate (<25), will be decreased in metabolic acidosis. The bicarbonate is being used-up to buffer the increasing levels of H^+ in the body, causing an eventual CO_2 deficit. **Please see the special topic on metabolic acidosis below for more details.** **Pattern:** 🌰 If the CO_2 is decreased (<25), along with an increased chloride (>106) and/or an increased anion gap (>12), metabolic acidosis is **probable**.

Metabolic Acidosis

In a metabolic acidosis, the body is in a state of increasing levels of H^+ ion. There are three main causes of H^+ increase:

1. **Direct administration or production of acid**- ammonium chloride supplementation, dietary acids, incomplete digestion of macronutrients, or aspirin use. Excess metabolic acids and ketones are produced during diabetic ketoacidosis. The CO_2 or bicarbonate level is decreased because it is being used up as a primary response to the build-up of excess acid.

2. **Base-losing acidosis** occurs in situations in which there is direct loss of bicarbonate from the small intestine. This is seen in conditions such as acute diarrhea, cholera, and chronic diarrhea. Bicarbonate is lost and the H^+ remains, causing a metabolic acidosis.

3. **Renal acidosis**- renal acidosis occurs during kidney failure. The kidney loses its ability to excrete H^+ due to the loss of renal tubular function. The remaining H^+ needs to be buffered and the body uses bicarbonate to do this, thus wasting the bicarbonate reserve.

Thiamine (vitamin B1) need	An increased anion gap (>12) is associated with thiamine deficiency. **Please see the special topic on thiamine deficiency on page 82 for more details.**
	Pattern:
	If CO_2 is decreased (<25) along with an increased anion gap (>12), thiamine deficiency is **possible.** Hemoglobin and Hematocrit levels may be normal or decreased (<37 or 0.37 in women and 40 or 0.4 in men). Due to thiamine's role in glycolysis, LDH levels (<140) may be decreased and glucose levels may be normal to increased (> 100 or 5.55 mmol/L).
Respiratory alkalosis	The CO_2 levels (<25) are often decreased in respiratory alkalosis, which is due to conditions that cause excess loss of CO_2 from the lungs. The classic presentation of this phenomenon is hyperventilation syndrome caused by hysteria, anxiety, stress, etc. Other causes include low blood pressure, shock, direct stimulation of the respiratory centers by drugs or trauma, and high altitude. Bicarbonate is lost due to the formation of CO_2 in the lungs.
Drug causes of ↓	❋ Salicylate excess (aspirin) ❋ Diuretics (chlorothiazide class)
Other conditions associated with ↓ levels include	Dehydration Diabetes Sleep apnea or shallow breathing Renal dysfunction Highly refined diet

"Chemical Sciatica"

An acidic neuritis can develop with an underlying chemical imbalance causing the build-up of lactic and pyruvic acids on a major nerve distribution. In the cranial nerves this can cause an increased sense of taste, smell or hearing. Commonly this may affect the distribution of the sciatic nerve and presents as "chemical sciatica". Consider "chemical sciatica" when structural causes have been ruled-out, particularly if the patient is obese, on a highly refined diet or deficient in Kreb's cycle nutrients (thiamine, magnesium, potassium). The following lab pattern may be reflective of this problem:

$$\downarrow CO_2 \; \downarrow Calcium \; \uparrow Chloride \; and \; \uparrow Anion \; gap$$

Eliminate all refined carbohydrates, alcohol, and high glycemic index foods and provide appropriate mineral and B-vitamin support, especially thiamine.

Related Tests:

Blood gases, serum chloride, potassium, sodium, and anion gap

Anion Gap

Background

The anion gap is the measurement of the difference between the sum of the serum cations (sodium and potassium) and the sum of the serum anions (CO_2/bicarbonate and chloride).

Discussion

 The difference reflects the concentrations of other extracellular anions, such as phosphates, sulfates, ketones, proteins and lactic acid. An increase in these unmeasured anions is associated with acidosis.

- An increased anion gap is associated with increased sodium and/or potassium and a decreased CO_2 and/or chloride.

- A decreased anion gap is associated with decreased sodium and/or potassium and an increased CO_2 and/or chloride.

- The anion gap is calculated by determining the difference between the sum of sodium and potassium and the sum of chloride and CO_2/bicarbonate.

Anion Gap = (Sodium + Potassium) - (Chloride + CO₂)

Ranges:

	Standard U.S. Units	**Standard International Units**
Conventional Laboratory Range	6 – 16 mEq/L	6 – 16 mmol/L
Optimal Range	7 – 12 mEq/L	7 – 12 mmol/L
Alarm Ranges	<4 or >25 mEq/L	<4 or >25 mmol/L

When would you run this test?

1. As a general measure of tissue acidity or alkalinity

Clinical implications

HIGH

Clinical Implication	Additional information
Thiamine (vitamin B1) need	An increased anion gap (>12) is associated with thiamine deficiency. **Please see the special topic on thiamine deficiency below for more details.** **Pattern:** If the anion gap is increased (>12) along with a decreased CO_2 (<25), thiamine deficiency is **possible**. Hemoglobin and hematocrit levels may be normal or decreased (<37 or 0.37 in women and 40 or 0.4 in men). Due to thiamine's role in glycolysis, LDH levels may be decreased and glucose levels may be normal to increased (> 100 or 5.55 mmol/L).

Thiamine Deficiency

Many indicators may be present with a thiamine need.

- Hypoglycemia
- Low blood pressure
- Chronic HCL need
- Carbohydrate sensitivity

- PMS
- Cyclic personality
- Anxiety
- Excess Alcohol, Drugs, or refined foods

- Thiamine deficiency can be assessed by checking red blood cell transketolase levels. RBC transketolase is an enzyme that cannot be produced in the absence or deficit of thiamine. It is an expensive test, so check for a decreased CO_2, an increased anion gap, and a low normal HCT and HGB first.

- It is well known that oral contraceptives will deplete many B-vitamins including thiamine and folate.

- If a chronic need for thiamine is present, consider that there may be an additional need for manganese, zinc, magnesium, and essential fatty acids, which are important co-factors for thiamine metabolism.

- It has been noted that people with a chronic need for thiamine may have a heavy metal body burden, particularly mercury, which interferes with thiamine and its role in the Kreb's cycle.

Metabolic Acidosis	An anion gap occurs in metabolic acidosis due to the excess metabolic acids and the increased serum chloride levels. CO_2, or bicarbonate, will be decreased in metabolic acidosis. The bicarbonate is being used up to buffer the increasing levels of H^+ in the body, causing an eventual CO_2 deficit. **Please see the special topic on metabolic acidosis on page 78 for more details.** **Pattern:** If the anion gap is increased (>12) along with a decreased CO_2 (<25) and an increased chloride (>106), metabolic acidosis is **probable**.

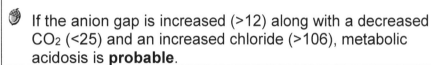

To receive master copies of our tracking forms and conversion tables please visit:

www.BloodChemistryAnalysis.com

If you're interested in a software program to help with your analysis please visit:
www.BloodChemSoftware.com

Drug causes of ↑	✳ Aspirin ✳ Diuretics ✳ Penicillin family of antibiotics	✳ Also rule out toxins such as Methanol, Ethylene Glycol, Gold, and other heavy metals
Other conditions associated with increased anion gap levels include	Dehydration Toxin ingestion	✳ Diabetes ✳ Lactic acidosis ✳ Metabolic acidosis

LOW

A decreased anion gap has been associated with multiple myeloma. It has been hypothesized that most calculated anion gaps are a result of laboratory error.

Clinical Implication	Additional information	
Conditions associated with decreased anion gap levels include	Lithium toxicity Increased serum Calcium and/or Magnesium	Multiple myeloma Neoplasm

Interfering Factors:

Falsely increased levels	Falsely decreased levels

• Anything that falsely decreases chloride or CO_2, or falsely increases sodium or potassium:
 	
   o Hemolyzed blood – K+ levels are elevated up to 50% of normal with even moderate hemolysis. Making a fist ten times with a tourniquet in place alone may result in an increased level of 10-20%, resulting in a ↓ anion gap
 	
• Excessive intake of licorice (herbal)
	• Anything that falsely increases chloride or CO_2, or falsely decreases sodium or potassium:
	
	   o Readings in infants
	
	   o Many drugs (Heparin, laxatives, sulphates, etc.)
	
	• High triglycerides or low protein levels can cause artificially low sodium levels resulting in an increased anion gap

Related Tests:

Serum sodium, potassium, CO_2, and chloride

Total Protein

Background

Total serum protein is composed of albumin and total globulin. Conditions that affect albumin and total globulin readings will impact the total protein value. A normal total protein is possible even if the albumin or globulin levels are abnormal, for example a condition that causes a decreased albumin and an increased globulin level will result in a normal total serum protein.

Discussion

 Protein absorption is affected by stomach, pancreatic, or small intestine dysfunction; as such, serum protein can be used to screen for nutritional deficiencies and functional digestive problems.

- A decreased total protein can be an indication of malnutrition, digestive dysfunction due to HCl need, or liver dysfunction. Malnutrition leads to a decreased total protein level in the serum primarily from lack of available essential amino acids.

- As the total protein level is composed of both albumin and total globulin levels an increased protein level must have a concomitant rise in one or more of these values. It is more likely to be an increase in the globulin fraction than the albumin level, unless there is dehydration that is causing the relative albumin increase.

Ranges:

	Standard U.S. Units	Standard International Units
Conventional Laboratory Range	6.0 – 8.5 g/dL	60 – 85g/L
Optimal Range	6.9 – 7.4 g/dL	69 – 74 g/L
Alarm Ranges	< 5.9 or > 8.5 g/dL	< 59 or > 85 g/L

When would you run this test?

1. To screen for nutritional deficiencies
2. To screen for functional digestive problems
3. To screen for dehydration

Clinical implications

HIGH

Clinical Implication	Additional information
Dehydration	If total protein is increased (>7.4 or 74 g/L) suspect dehydration. Dehydration is a very common problem and should be factored into your blood chemistry and CBC analysis. **Please see special topic on page 90 for more details.** **Pattern:** 🌰 Suspect a short-term (acute) dehydration if there is an increased HGB (>14.5 or 145 in women or 15 or 150 in men) and/or HCT (>44 or 0.44 in women and >48 or 0.48 in men) along with an increased RBC count (>4.5 in women and >4.9 in men). A relative increase in sodium (>142) and potassium (>4.5) can be noted as well. 🌰 Suspect a long-term (chronic) dehydration if any of the above findings are accompanied by an increased albumin (>5.0 or 50 g/L), increased BUN (>16 or 5.71 mmol/L), and/or serum protein (>7.4 or 74 g/L).
Other conditions associated with increased total protein levels include	🌰 Adrenal Hypofunction ✳ Diabetes 🌰 Liver/Biliary dysfunction ✳ Neoplasm 🌰 Amino Acid need ✳ Rheumatoid arthritis

LOW

Clinical Implication	Additional information
Hypochlorhydria	A decreased or normal total protein level is often associated with a decreased production of hydrochloric acid in the stomach (Hypochlorhydria). **Please see the special topic on hypochlorhydria on page 96 for more details.** **Pattern:** Hypochlorhydria is **possible** with an increased globulin level (>2.8 or 28 g/L) and a normal or decreased total protein (6.9 or 69 g/L) and/or albumin (< 4.0 or 40 g/L). Hypochlorhydria is **probable** if globulin levels are increased (>2.8 or 28 g/L) along with an increased BUN (>16 or 5.71 mmol/L), a decreased or normal total protein (6.9 or 69 g/L) and/or albumin (<4.0 or 40 g/L), and/or decreased serum

	phosphorous (<3.0 or <0.97 mmol/L).
	Other values that may be reflective of a developing or chronic hypochlorhydria include increased or decreased gastrin (<50 or >100), an increased MCV (>90) and MCH (>31.9), a decreased or normal calcium (<9.2 or 2.3 mmol/L) and iron (50 or 8.96 μmol/dL), a decreased CO_2 (<25), an increased anion gap (>12) and a decreased alkaline phosphatase (<70)
	Some of clinical indications of Hypochlorhydria include:
	1. Gas and bloating shortly after meals 2. Sense of fullness/ Easy satiety 3. Nausea after taking supplements 4. Weak, peeling, or cracked nails 5. Dilated capillaries in cheeks and nose in non-alcoholics
Digestive dysfunction/ inflammation	Suspect primary digestive inflammation or inflammation secondary to HCL insufficiency with a low total protein (6.9 or 69 g/L). This pattern will be similar to that of Hypochlorhydria but the globulin may be decreased (< 2.4 or 24 g/L) unless inflammation is severe. Many patients with the subjective and laboratory indications of HCl need experience an aggravation of their symptoms when taking HCL supplementation. Patients with this type of reaction probably have gastric inflammation due to a long-term HCL need. If inflammation is suspected or present, support the digestive terrain to heal the inflammation appropriately for 3 to 4 weeks prior to initiating HCl therapy. Acute digestive inflammation may lead to an increased globulin level (>2.8 or 28 g/L) due to the increased production of inflammatory immunoglobulins. Chronic digestive inflammation due to colitis, enteritis, Crohn's, etc. will compromise protein breakdown and absorption, leading to a widespread protein deficiency in the body and a decreased level of the inflammatory immunoglobulins, hence the decreased total globulin level (<2.4 or 24 g/L). **Pattern**: Decreased total globulin (<2.4 or 24 g/L), decreased serum phosphorous (<3.0 or 0.97 mmol/L) , increased BUN (>16 or 5.71 mmol/L) , basophils (>1) and ESR.
Liver dysfunction	Dysfunction in the liver will have a great impact on protein production and synthesis, which will affect total serum protein

	levels. Therefore, a decreased total serum protein level (<6.9 or 69 g/L) may be indicative of a liver dysfunction. Functionally oriented liver problems, such as detoxification issues, liver congestion, and conjugation problems are extremely common and should be evaluated based upon early prognostic indicators. The liver should always be viewed in the context of the hepato-biliary tree. Some of the key clinical indicators include: 1. Pain between shoulder blades 2. Stomach upset by greasy foods 3. If drinking alcohol, easily intoxicated 4. Headache over the eye 5. Sensitive to chemicals (perfume, cleaning solvents, insecticides, exhaust, etc.) 6. Hemorrhoids or varicose veins
Diet- Low protein Malnutrition/ amino acid need	Protein digestion is dependent on an optimal pH in the stomach. A decreased total protein (<6.9 or 69 g/L) can be an indicator for digestive dysfunction, which will greatly compromise protein digestion and absorption. Protein malnutrition is due primarily to the lack of available essential amino acids from the diet.
Other conditions associated with decreased total protein levels include	Thyroid hyperfunction CHF Adrenal hyperfunction Hypertension Thiamine deficiency Renal dysfunction Posterior pituitary dysfunction

Interfering Factors:

Falsely increased levels	Falsely decreased levels
• Hemolysis and dehydration will elevate the serum protein	• Normal during pregnancy, particularly during 3rd trimester or with any condition with prolonged bed rest

Related Tests:

Albumin, total globulin, liver enzymes, WBC w/ differential, serum protein electrophoresis, Serum Gastrin, IgA, IgM, IgG, HCT, HGB

Albumin

Background

Albumin is one of the major blood proteins. Produced primarily in the liver, it plays a major role in water distribution and serves as a transport protein for hormones and various drugs. Albumin is responsible for about 80% of the colloid-osmotic pressure between blood and tissue fluids.

Discussion

 Albumin levels are affected by digestive dysfunction and a decreased albumin can be an indication of malnutrition, digestive dysfunction due to HCl need, or liver dysfunction. Malnutrition leads to a decreased albumin level in the serum primarily from lack of available essential amino acids.

- Serum albumin levels and its production are greatly affected by the health and function of the liver, because albumin is produced almost entirely by the liver. Liver dysfunction will cause a decreased albumin level.

- When albumin is decreased, osmotic pressure is disturbed and fluid can leak into intracellular spaces, leading to edema.

- Decreased albumin can be a strong indicator of a frank or developing oxidative stress and excess free radical activity.

Ranges:

	Standard U.S. Units	Standard International Units
Conventional Laboratory Range	3.5 – 5.5 g/dL	35 – 55 g/L
Optimal Range	4.0 – 5.0 g/dL	40 – 50 g/L
Alarm Ranges	< 4.0 g/dL	< 40 g/L

When would you run this test?

1. To ascertain digestive sufficiency
2. To screen for hydration

Clinical implications

HIGH

Clinical Implication	Additional information
Dehydration	If albumin is increased (>5.0 or 50 g/L) suspect dehydration. Dehydration is a very common problem and should be factored into your blood chemistry and CBC analysis. **Please see special topic below for more details.** **Pattern:** 🌰 Suspect a short-term (acute) dehydration if there is an increased HGB (>14.5 or 145 in women or 15 or 150 in men) and/or HCT (>44 or 0.44 in women and >48 or 0.48 in men) along with an increased RBC count (>4.5 in women and >4.9 in men). A relative increase in sodium (>142) and potassium (>4.5) can be noted as well. 🌰 Suspect a long-term (chronic) dehydration if any of the above findings are accompanied by an increased albumin (>5.0 or 50 g/L) , increased BUN (>16 or 5.71 mmol/L)and/or serum protein (>7.4 or 74 g/L).

Dehydration

Insufficient water is the most common cause of dehydration and is endemic to the population. Almost every fluid, with the exception of water and most non-diuretic botanical teas, causes dehydration. Notably, caffeine, alcohol, carbonated beverages,and juices can actually "rob" the body of water and needed electrolytes. Water is the single most important nutrient for optimal biochemistry and functioning.

Pure or filtered water is best to ensure proper hydration without the risk of unnecessary contaminants. One can approximate ½ of their body weight in pounds to their daily needed amount of water in ounces. Extra water intake is required during periods of elevated water loss (sweating, vomiting, diarrhea, and diuretic intake.) Even on an average day, the human body loses 2 ½ liters of water with normal physiological activity. The lungs alone expel 12% of this volume.

 Both dehydration and over-hydration put significant stress on the kidneys. Adequate hydration is necessary for basic chemistry reactions, digestion, electrolyte balance, hormone transport, renal and cardiac function.

If you suspect dehydration from history, clinical findings or a blood chemistry screen, evaluate for diuretic use and adequate intake. Over the counter and prescription drugs, botanical medicines, caffeine etc. re common findings.

Other conditions associated with increased albumin levels include	Thyroid hypofunction	Adrenal hypofunction

LOW

Clinical Implication	Additional information
Hypochlorhydria	A decreased albumin level (<4.0 or 40g/L) is often associated with a decreased production of hydrochloric acid in the stomach (hypochlorhydria). **Please see the special topic on hypochlorhydria on page 96 for more details.** **Pattern:** Hypochlorhydria is **possible** with an increased globulin level (>2.8 or 28 g/L) and a normal or decreased total protein (<6.9 or 69 g/L) and/or albumin (<4.0 or 40g/L). Hypochlorhydria is **probable** if globulin levels are increased (>2.8 or 28 g/L) along with an increased BUN (>16 or 5.71 mmol/L), a decreased or normal total protein (<6.9 or 69 g/L) and/or albumin (<4.0 or 40g/L) and/or decreased serum phosphorous (<3.0 or <0.97 mmol/L). Other values that may be reflective of a developing or chronic hypochlorhydria include increased or decreased gastrin (<50 or >100), an increased MCV (>90) and MCH (>31.9), a decreased or normal calcium (<9.2 or 2.3 mmol/L) and iron (<50 or 8.96μmol/dL), a decreased chloride (<100), an increased anion gap (>12) and a decreased alkaline phosphatase (<70). Some of clinical indications of Hypochlorhydria include: 1. Gas and bloating shortly after meals 2. Sense of fullness/ Easy satiety 3. Nausea after taking supplements 4. Weak, peeling, or cracked nails 5. Dilated capillaries in cheeks and nose in non-alcoholics
Liver dysfunction	Albumin is produced almost entirely by the liver and dysfunction in the liver will have a great impact on albumin production and serum albumin levels. Therefore, a decreased albumin level may be indicative of a liver dysfunction that prevents the synthesis and formation of protein. A decreased

91

	albumin (<4.0 or 40g/L) may be observed before any changes in liver enzymes are noted.
	Functionally oriented liver problems, such as detoxification issues, liver congestion and conjugation problems are extremely common and should be evaluated based upon early prognostic indicators. The liver should always be viewed in the context of the hepato-biliary tree. Some of the key clinical indicators include:
	1. Pain between shoulder blades
	2. Stomach upset by greasy foods
	3. If drinking alcohol, easily intoxicated
	4. Headache over the eye
	5. Sensitive to chemicals (perfume, cleaning solvents, insecticides, exhaust, etc.)
	6. Hemorrhoids or varicose veins
Oxidative stress and excess Free Radical Activity	Suspect excess free radical activity and oxidative stress if the albumin is decreased.
	Pattern:
	If albumin levels are decreased (<4.0 or 40g/L) along with a decreased lymphocyte count (<20), a total cholesterol that is suddenly below its historical level, an increased total globulin (>2.8 or 28 g/L) an increased uric acid (>5.9 or > 351 µmol/dL) and low platelet levels (<150), free radical pathology, which increases the risk for developing a neoplasm, should be investigated. This can be accomplished in the office using the Oxidata free radical test. **Please see page 152 for a discussion of this test.** Oxidative stress can cause an increased destruction of red blood cells; in these situations you will see an elevated bilirubin level (>1.2 or 20.5 µmol/dL).
	Other tests include: Acid Phosphatase, serum protein electrophoresis, CEA, Anti-malignin Antibody, HCG, Alpha Fetoprotein, etc. If Alpha 1, Alpha 2, or gamma globulins are increased on a serum protein electrophoresis, free radical pathology should be investigated immediately.
Vitamin C need	A decreased albumin level is associated with vitamin C need.
	Pattern:
	🍁 Albumin will frequently be decreased (<4.0 or 40g/L) along a decreased HCT (<37 or 0.37 in women and 40 or 0.4 in men), HGB (<13.5 or 135 g/L in women and <14 or 140 in men), MCH (<28), MCHC (<32), and serum iron (< 50 or 8.96µmol/dL). There will also be an increased MCV (>90),

	alkaline phosphatase (>100), and fibrinogen.
	Both the lingual ascorbic acid test and urinary vitamin C will generally be out of range.
	Please see the special topic on the lingual ascorbic acid test on page 218 for more details.
Pregnancy	A decreased albumin reading (<4.0 or 40g/L) is normal in pregnancy.
	Please see the special topic on Pregnancy and its impact on Laboratory Values on page 94 for more details
Other conditions associated with decreased albumin levels include	Immune insufficiency Hemorrhage Protein malnutrition Liver cirrhosis Thyroid hyperfunction Alcoholism B12/Folate deficiency anemia Hypocalcemia

Interfering Factors:

Falsely increased levels	Falsely decreased levels
• Dehydration	• Excessive hemolysis in patient sample taken supine

Related Tests:

Albumin/globulin ratio, total protein, total globulin, serum protein electrophoresis (SPE), liver enzymes, WBC and differential, alpha 1 glycoproteins, CEA and other tests used to confirm neoplasm.

Pregnancy and its impact on Laboratory values

Pregnancy presents an interesting challenge when doing blood chemistry and CBC analysis. The demands placed upon the body's normal physiology and biochemistry during this period of rapid growth and development will cause many of the values to be outside of their optimal level. This should not necessarily be viewed as indicative of a disease process. The following represents some of the "normal" changes associated with pregnancy.

Throughout Pregnancy

⬇ Albumin

⬆ Serum cholesterol, LDL and triglycerides

⬆ Blood glucose

⬇ HGB and HCT

⬆ MCV and MCH

⬇ RBC

⬇ T-3 uptake

⬆ T-4 (2nd and 3rd trimester)

⬇ Total protein

⬇ Uric acid

⬇ Creatinine

⬇ BUN

⬆ Alkaline phosphatase

⬇ SGOT

⬆ ESR (2nd and 3rd trimester)

Late Pregnancy (3rd trimester)

⬇ lymphocytes

⬆ Neutrophils

⬆ Total WBCs

⬇ Calcium

⬇ Total protein

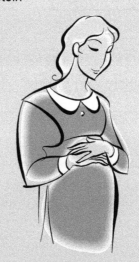

Total Globulin

Background

Total serum globulin is composed of individual globulin fractions called alpha 1, alpha 2, beta and gamma fractions. The total globulin level is greatly impacted by concomitant increases or decreases in one or more of these fractions. Globulins function to transport substances in the blood and constitute the antibody system, clotting proteins and complement. Globulins are produced in the liver, the reticuloendothelial system, and other tissues.

Discussion

Care must be taken when making a diagnosis based upon the total globulin alone because total globulin is composed of 4 different fractions. Inflammatory, degenerative, or infectious processes are associated with an increased production of antibodies. The total serum globulin is a useful way to assess these processes, as many antibodies are synthesized from globulins.

● With accompanying subjective indicators, a total globulin can help to confirm an underlying digestive problem of an inflammatory or infectious nature. Secretory IgA levels are often decreased in these situations.

● A serum protein electrophoresis should be completed when the total serum globulin exceeds 3.5 or drops below 2.0 g/100 mL. Protein electrophoresis is an excellent method of identifying the specific globulin that is responsible for the total serum globulin increase or decrease.

Ranges:

	Standard U.S. Units	Standard International Units
Conventional Laboratory Range	2.0 – 3.9 g/dL	20 – 39 g/L
Optimal Range	2.4 - 2.8 g/dL	24 – 28 g/L
Alarm Ranges	< 2.0 or > 3.5 g/dL	<20 or > 35 g/L

When would you run this test?

1. To investigate inflammatory and/or immunological disturbances
2. To ascertain digestive sufficiency

Clinical implications

HIGH

Clinical Implication	Additional information
Hypochlorhydria	An increased total globulin level is often associated with a decreased production of hydrochloric acid in the stomach (hypochlorhydria). Please see the special topic on hypochlorhydria below for more details. **Pattern**: Hypochlorhydria is **possible** with an increased globulin level (>2.8 or 28 g/L) and a normal or decreased total protein (<6.9 or 69 g/L). Hypochlorhydria is **probable** if globulin levels are increased (>2.8 or 28 g/L) along with an increased BUN (>16 or 5.71 mmol/L), a decreased or normal total protein (<6.9 or 69 g/L) and/or albumin (<4.0 or 40g/L) and/or decreased serum phosphorous (<3.0 or <0.97 mmol/L). Other values that may be reflective of a developing or chronic hypochlorhydria include increased or decreased gastrin (<50 or >100), an increased MCV (>90) and MCH (>31.9), a decreased or normal calcium (<9.2 or 2.3 mmol/L) and Iron (< 50 or 8.96μmol/dL), a decreased chloride (<100), an increased anion gap (>12) and a decreased alkaline phosphatase (<70). Some of clinical indications of Hypochlorhydria include: 1. Gas and bloating shortly after meals 2. Sense of fullness/ Easy satiety 3. Nausea after taking supplements 4. Weak, peeling, or cracked nails 5. Dilated capillaries in cheeks and nose in non-alcoholics

Digestive Insufficiency- Hypochlorhydria

Hypochlorhydria, or the insufficient production of stomach acid, is a very common clinical problem with influences far beyond the digestive tract (i.e. food and environmental sensitivity, asthma, intestinal parasites, dermatological problems, autoimmune disease and arthralgias.)

Many factors contribute to the development of chronic hypochlorhydria including:

- Poor food choices (Standard American Diet)
- Excess carbohydrate consumption (depletes critical co-factors)
- Insufficient protein stimulation (veganism, low protein diets)
- Sympathetic dominance/stress (inhibits the parasympathetic control of digestive secretions)
- Zinc and thiamine deficiencies (essential to the production of HCL)
- Antacid use (temporary symptom relief/worsens problem)
- Alcohol and NSAID use (lead to gastric atrophy)

The inability to produce HCl is frequently due to a need for **chloride** (low serum chloride) or a need for **zinc** (ALP will generally be decreased) and **thiamine** (CO_2 will generally be decreased with an increased anion gap). These are primary nutritional factors required for the synthesis of hydrochloric acid. Paradoxically, sufficient HCL is needed in order to properly absorb these nutrients as well. Hence, the chronic nature of this problem is often perpetuated.

When hypochlorhydria is present, pancreatic and biliary dysfunction are generally also present, secondary to the need for HCl. If the food bolus is not acid enough upon exiting the stomach, it will not trigger CCK properly and stimulate pancreatic enzyme production and release. The subsequent improperly digested proteins and carbohydrates contribute to the growth of opportunistic organisms and often lead to a dysbiotic intestinal tract. Checking urinary indican levels is an excellent means for determining protein putrefaction, carbohydrate fermentation, and dysbiotic activity.

Hydrochloric acid supplementation is often fundamental to breaking this cycle of chronic digestive insufficiency. Short term administration stimulates the body's own eventual production of HCL by reducing the tremendous digestive stress upon an otherwise compromised gut mucosa.

Liver damage/infections	Increased levels of total globulin (>2.8 or 28 g/L) are often seen in conditions such as hepatitis, fatty liver, or cirrhosis. The body produces increased levels of immunoglobulins in response to tissue and cellular damage, destruction, or infection. Rule out liver problem or infection SGPT/ALT, SGOT/AST, GGTP, and serum protein electrophoresis. Consider fatty liver in obese patients or those with elevated lipids. Rule out cirrhosis if elevated in conjunction with liver enzyme abnormalities.
Oxidative Stress and Free Radical Activity	Suspect excess free radical activity and oxidative stress if the total globulin level is increased.

	Pattern: If the total globulin level is increased (>2.8 or 28 g/L) along with a total cholesterol level that is suddenly below its historical level and a decreased lymphocyte count (<20), a decreased albumin (<4.0 or 40 g/L) and a decreased platelet level (<150) free radical pathology, which increases the risk for developing a neoplasm, should be investigated. This can be accomplished in the office using the Oxidata free radical test. **Please see page 152 for a discussion of this test.** Oxidative stress can cause an increased destruction of red blood cells; in these situations you will see an elevated bilirubin level (>1.2 or 20.5 µmol/dL). Other tests include: Acid Phosphatase, serum protein Electrophoresis, CEA, Anti-malignin Antibody, HCG, Alpha Fetoprotein, etc. If Alpha 1, Alpha 2, or gamma globulins are increased on a serum protein electrophoresis, free radical pathology should be investigated immediately.
Heavy metal/ Chemical toxicity	Chronic levels of chemical and/or heavy metal toxicity can lead to an elevation in total globulins due to the persistent low-level tissue inflammation.
Immune Activation	The total globulin level constitutes the body's antibody system. It is composed of four fractions (alpha 1, alpha 2, beta and gamma globulin). An increased level of total globulins (>2.8 or 28 g/L) can therefore indicate an increase in one or more of these fractions that has been activated due to an infectious or inflammatory process. Many auto-immune conditions will first present with this pattern.
Other conditions associated with increased Globulin levels include	Parasites (intestinal or liver) Rheumatoid arthritis Auto-immune processes Tissue destruction Exogenous hormone administration Acute viral/bacterial infections (Hepatitis)

LOW

Clinical Implication	Additional information
Digestive Dysfunction Inflammation	Suspect primary digestive inflammation or inflammation secondary to HCL insufficiency. The pattern will be similar to that of hypochlorhydria but the globulin may be decreased (< 2.4 or 24 g/L) unless inflammation is severe. Many patients with the subjective and laboratory indications of HCl need experience an aggravation of their symptoms when

	taking HCL supplementation. Patiens with this type of reaction probably have gastric inflammation due to a long-term HCL need. If inflammation is suspected or present, support the digestive terrain to heal the inflammation appropriately for 3 to 4 weeks prior to initiating HCl therapy.
	Acute digestive inflammation may lead to an increased globulin level (>2.8 or 28 g/L) due to the increased production of inflammatory immunoglobulins. Chronic digestive inflammation due to colitis, enteritis, Crohn's etc., will compromise protein breakdown and absorption, leading to a widespread protein deficiency in the body and a decreased level of the inflammatory immunoglobulins, hence the decreased total globulin level (<2.4 or 24 g/L).
	Pattern:
	Decreased total globulin (<2.4 or 24 g/L), decreased serum phosphorous (<3.0 or <0.97 mmol/L), increased BUN (>16 or 5.71 mmol/L), basophils (> 1) and ESR.
Immune insufficiency	A decreased total globulin (< 2.0 or 20 g/L) suggests immune insufficiency. Suspect an increased use of globulin by the liver, spleen, thymus, kidneys, or heart. Apart from known kidney or heart dysfunction, rule out a chronic immune disruptor (virus, xenobiotics, toxicity etc.) and consider a serum protein electrophoresis test (look for a decreased gamma fraction) in the investigation of immune insufficiency.
Other conditions associated with decreased globulin levels include	Anemia Liver Disease Chronic viral/bacterial infections

Interfering Factors:

Falsely increased levels	Falsely decreased levels
• none noted	• none noted

Related Tests:
Albumin, A/G ratio, total protein, serum protein electrophoresis (SPE), serum Gastrin, liver enzymes, sedimentation rate, WBC and differential, alpha I Glycoproteins, CEA, and other tests used to confirm neoplasm.

Albumin/Globulin Ratio

Background

The albumin/globulin ratio is dependent on the albumin and total globulin levels. It should be used as a rough guide, due to the variability in albumin and globulin levels, and should always be viewed in context with globulin and albumin. The globulin portion of the ratio is the most clinically relevant and can have the most impact.

Discussion

 An increased ratio, which is fairly uncommon, is usually due to either a decreased globulin or an increased albumin level, a situation that is usually due to dehydration.

- A decreased ratio is usually due to either an albumin decrease with a globulin increase or a normal albumin with a greatly increased globulin. The former is more common.

- A decreased ratio is often called a suppressed, low or reversed ratio and is generally considered a reflection of liver dysfunction, as both a decreased albumin and an increased globulin can be caused by liver dysfunction.

Ranges:

	Standard U.S. Units	Standard International Units
Conventional Laboratory Range	1.1 – 2.5	1.1 – 2.5
Optimal Range	1.5 – 2.0	1.5 – 2.0
Alarm Ranges	< 1.0	< 1.0

When would you run this test?

1. To investigate inflammatory and/or immunological disturbances
2. To ascertain digestive sufficiency

Clinical implications

HIGH

Clinical Implication	Additional information	
Other conditions associated with increased albumin/globulin ratio levels include	Thyroid hypofunction (↑ Albumin) Adrenal hypofunction (↑ Albumin)	Blood viscosity may be too high due to blood stasis

LOW

Clinical Implication	Additional information
Liver dysfunction	Liver dysfunction will cause a decreased albumin level (<4.0 or 40g/L) and an increased globulin level (>2.8 or 28 g/L), both of which will cause a decreased albumin/globulin ratio. Functionally oriented liver problems, such as detoxification issues, liver congestion, and conjugation problems are extremely common and should be evaluated based upon early prognostic indicators. The liver should always be viewed in the context of the hepato-biliary tree. Some of the key clinical indicators include: 1. Pain between shoulder blades 2. Stomach upset by greasy foods 3. If drinking alcohol, easily intoxicated 4. Headache over the eye 5. Sensitive to chemicals (perfume, cleaning solvents, insecticides, exhaust, etc.) 6. Hemorrhoids or varicose veins
Immune Activation	Another cause of a decreased albumin/globulin ratio is a low normal albumin with an increased globulin. The total globulin level constitutes the body's antibody system. It is composed of four fractions (alpha 1, alpha 2, beta and gamma globulin). An increased level of total globulins can therefore indicate an increase in one or more of these fractions that has been activated due to an infectious or inflammatory process. Many auto-immune conditions will first present with this pattern.
Other conditions associated with decreased albumin/globulin levels include	Blood too thin (rule out chronic aspirin use, unnecessary blood thinners)

Interfering Factors:

Falsely increased levels	Falsely decreased levels
• Dehydration	• Normal during pregnancy
	• Excessive hemolysis in patient sample taken supine

Related Tests:

Albumin, total globulin, serum protein electrophoresis (SPE), alpha 1, alpha 2, beta and gamma globulin, liver enzymes.

Serum Calcium

Background

The majority of the calcium in the body (98-99%) is stored in the bone and teeth, which act as a major functional store. The body will use this reservoir to maintain the calcium blood levels, which are tightly regulated within a narrow range. Serum Calcium exists in three different forms in the plasma:

1. 40% of the calcium in the plasma is combined with plasma proteins such as albumin and is non-diffusible through the cell membrane. It is therefore important to know the serum albumin level to interpret calcium levels.

2. 10% of the calcium in the plasma is combined to other substances, such as phosphate and citrate, and is freely diffusible through the cell membrane

3. The remaining 50% of the plasma calcium is in the ionized form and is freely diffusible through the cellular membrane.

Approximately half of the plasma calcium is in an ionic form. This ionic calcium is the only form of calcium that can be used by the body for its many physiological and metabolic functions: muscle contraction, blood clotting, cardiac function, and transmission of nerve impulses to name a few.

Calcium absorption is dependent on an optimal acidity of the stomach. It is also affected by the amount of phosphate and magnesium present. Actual absorption occurs in the upper part of the small intestine. Calcium affects the amount of protein absorption and helps move fats through the intestinal wall.

Ionized calcium levels are regulated by parathyroid hormone (PTH) and vitamin D. Produced by the parathyroid gland, PTH is the most important hormone in calcium regulation. It promotes bone resorption to increase serum calcium by activating osteoclasts, it increases the reabsorption of calcium from the urine, promotes the activation of the active form of vitamin D (Cholecalciferol,) and enhances the absorption of calcium from the intestine.

Discussion

 Ionized calcium is required for the biochemistry of inflammation and tissue repair, particularly the leukocytes for phagocytosis. It is a vital component of the interstitial matrix facilitating cell to cell adhesion and communication, and provides cell membrane stability. Calcium is also important in vascular integrity and clotting, and bone metabolism.

- There is a predominant belief that calcium deficiency is very common and that most patients would benefit from daily supplementation. Clinical experience suggests that a calcium need has less to do with calcium deficiency and more to do with an inability to absorb and utilize dietary calcium. Rule out hypochlorhydria, the need for magnesium, phosphorous, vitamin A, B and C, unsaturated fatty acids, and iodine as some of the reasons for a "calcium" need, before supplementing with calcium.

- When subjective indicators or lab testing identify a potential calcium need, the lack of synergistic co-factors that aid in calcium metabolism is often the main problem. Please see the special topic on calcium co-factors below for more detail.

Common subjective indications of calcium need are:

1. Muscle cramps at rest
2. Frequent nose bleeds
3. Soft fingernails
4. Frequent cold sores, skin rashes, sunburn or hives
5. High or low blood pressure.
6. Irritability
7. Fever with a mild cold or virus
8. Frequent hoarseness

Ranges:

	Standard U.S. Units	Standard International Units
Conventional Laboratory Range	8.5 – 10.8 mg/dL	2.13 – 2.70 mmol/L
Optimal Range	9.2 – 10.0 mg/dL	2.30 – 2.50 mmol/L
Alarm Ranges	< 7.0 or > 12.0 mg/dL	< 1.75 or > 3.00 mmol/L

When would you run this test?

1. To assess parathyroid function
2. To ascertain digestive sufficiency

 # Urinary Calcium "Sulkowitch" Test

Urinary calcium levels closely correlate with serum calcium. Checking urinary calcium levels with the Sulkowitch test can be very helpful anytime the serum calcium levels are increased or decreased. It can be used to monitor whether or not the calcium levels are returning to normal.

Clinical implications

HIGH

Clinical Implication	Additional information
Parathyroid Hyperfunction	Parathyroid hyperfunction will cause an increase in PTH levels, which can lead to significantly increased serum calcium.
	Pattern:
	If the serum calcium is significantly increased (>10.5 or 2.5 mmol/L) with a decreased phosphorous (<3.0 or <0.97 mmol/L) parathyroid hyperfunction is **possible**. Alkaline phosphatase levels may also be increased (>100), along with a normal or decreased serum or RBC magnesium.
	Follow-up with a serum parathyroid hormone test. If parathyroid hormone levels are also increased, presume clinical hyperparathyroidism exists.
	✤ Hyperparathyroidism may be due to space-occupying lesions on one or more of the glands. Surgical removal may be necessary to determine if there is a neoplasm.
	✤ A patient with increased serum calcium and an increased PTH should be checked by an endocrinologist, as hyperparathyroidism is a serious condition.
Thyroid hypofunction	Serum calcium may be increased in either primary thyroid hypofunction or secondary thyroid hypofunction due to anterior pituitary hypofunction.
	Pattern:
	◉ With primary hypothyroidism the calcium levels may be increased (>10.5 or 2.5 mmol/L) along with an increased TSH (>4.0)
	◉ With secondary thyroid hypofunction due to anterior pituitary hypofunction, the calcium levels may be increased (>10.5 or 2.5 mmol/L) along with a decreased TSH (<2.0).
Impaired cell membrane health	Increased serum levels of calcium (>10.5 or 2.5 mmol/L) can be suggestive of cellular membrane disruption and/or destruction as it is a vital component of the interstitial matrix, facilitating cell to cell adhesion and communication. Calcium will be released into the serum if this matrix is disrupted. Space-occupying lesions should be considered and ruled out with appropriate examination and testing.

Other conditions associated with increased calcium levels include	Ovarian hypofunction	Hypothalamic-pituitary axis dysfunction
	Vitamin D (excess ingestion)	Neoplasm
	Adrenal hypofunction	Epilepsy
	Poor fat emulsification	Osteoporosis

LOW

Before considering the clinical implications listed below, please check the serum albumin level to make sure that a decrease in serum albumin is not the cause for a relative serum calcium decrease, as much of the serum calcium is bound to albumin and this is the most common cause of a decreased calcium level.

For every decrease in albumin by 1 mg/dL, calcium should be corrected upward by 0.8 mg/dL.

Clinical Implication	Additional information
Parathyroid Hypofunction	Parathyroid hypofunction will lead to decreased PTH levels that can cause decreased serum calcium. **Pattern:** If calcium is decreased (<9.2 or 2.3 mmol/L) along with a high phosphorous level (>4.0 or 1.29 mmol/L), parathyroid hypofunction is **possible**. Alkaline phosphatase levels may also be normal or decreased (<70). Follow up with a serum parathyroid hormone test. If parathyroid hormone levels are also decreased presume clinical hypoparathyroidism exists.
Calcium need and/or a need for its co-factor	Calcium need is not just a matter of calcium supplementation. Calcium regulation is a game of co-factors. **Please see the special topic below for more information.**

Calcium Regulation- a need for co-factors

Calcium regulation in the body is determined by a number of different co-factors that are necessary for adequate digestion, absorption and utilization of calcium. These include:

Calcium Regulation- a need for co-factors

1. **Digestion**
   - Calcium and other minerals require Hydrochloric Acid (HCl) for uptake. Ensuring adequate stomach function can increase calcium absorption from the diet.

2. **Vitamin D**
   - Vitamin D acts to increase calcium levels in the blood by increasing calcium uptake from the gut, by pulling calcium from the tissue and decreasing fecal and urinary calcium loss

3. **Essential Fatty Acid**
   - Essential fatty acids help increase tissue calcium levels and are necessary for the transport of calcium across the cell membrane into the cells

4. **Systemic pH**
   - Calcium is a major buffer of blood pH and as such is affected by changes in blood pH.
   - When the blood becomes too alkaline, calcium precipitates out of solution and can be deposited in excess into inappropriate tissue:
     - Eyes—cataracts
     - Bones—bone spurs
     - Joints—bursitis
     - Kidneys—stones
   - When the blood becomes too acidic, calcium is resorbed from tissue, which can cause problems in the following areas:
     - Skin—cold sores, herpes, sunburn, canker sores, etc.
     - Teeth—dental caries, gum problems
     - Bones—osteoporosis

5. **Calcium must be in balance with the other macro minerals**
   - Phosphorous is the opposing acid mineral
   - Magnesium is often deficient in the American diet, and is important for the body to appropriately use calcium

6. **Trace minerals are also important in the utilization of Calcium:**
   - Manganese, boron, copper, zinc, potassium

7. **Hormones**
   Calcium metabolism is affected and regulated by a number of different hormones
   - **Parathyroid hormone (PTH)**

Calcium Regulation- a need for co-factors

- PTH increases serum Calcium levels by increasing calcium uptake from the gut, by pulling calcium from tissue, by decreasing urinary and fecal loss of calcium and by increasing osteoclastic activity in the bone.

- **Calcitonin**
  - Calcitonin is secreted from the thyroid gland and has a weak effect of blood calcium. It inhibits osteolytic activity of the osteoclasts and promotes calcium deposition in the bone, thereby decreasing blood calcium levels+

- **Sex hormones**
  - The sex hormones' effect on calcium metabolism is due to their effect on bone metabolism
  - Progesterone and estrogen promote bone building and therefore may lead to a decrease in serum calcium.
  - Testosterone promotes calcium retention in the bone and may cause a decrease in serum calcium.

| **Hypochlorhydria**
 | A decreased serum calcium is often associated with a decreased production of hydrochloric acid in the stomach (hypochlorhydria). **Please see the special topic on page 96 for more details on hypochlorhydria.**

Pattern:
Hypochlorhydria is **possible** with a decreased serum calcium (<9.2 or 2.3 mmol/L) and an increased or decreased globulin level (< 2.4 / 24 g/L or >2.8 / 28 g/L) and a normal or decreased total protein (<6.9 or 69 g/L).

Hypochlorhydria is **probable** if globulin levels are increased (>2.8 or 28 g/L) or decreased (<2.4 or 24 g/L) along with an increased BUN (>16 or 5.71 mmol/L), a decreased or normal total protein (<6.9 or 69 g/L) and/or albumin (<4.0 or 40g/L) and/or decreased serum phosphorous (<3.0 or <0.97 mmol/L).

Other values that may be reflective of a developing or chronic hypochlorhydria include increased or decreased gastrin (<50 or >100), an increased MCV (>90) and MCH (>31.9), a decreased or normal calcium (<9.2 or 2.3 mmol/L) and iron (< 50 or 8.96 μmol/dL), a decreased CO_2 (<25) an increased |

	anion gap (>12), and a decreased alkaline phosphatase (<70) Some of clinical indications of hypochlorhydria include: 1. Gas and bloating shortly after meals 2. Sense of fullness/ easy satiety 3. Nausea after taking supplements 4. Weak, peeling, or cracked nails 5. Dilated capillaries in cheeks and nose in non-alcoholics
Other conditions associated with decreased calcium levels include	Ovarian hypofunction Osteoporosis Vitamin D insufficiency Metabolic acidosis Protein malnutrition Poor fatty acid utilization

Calcium "Deficiency" or an abnormal Ca:Phos ratio?

A low calcium/phosphorous ratio favors the binding of calcium to phosphorous to form calcium phosphate. This will decrease the levels of ionized calcium.

A high calcium/phosphorous ratio favors deposition of calcium into the soft tissue. This deposition will decrease the availability of ionized calcium and reduce the serum calcium reading.

Interfering Factors:

Falsely increased levels	Falsely decreased levels
• Thiazide diuretics (impair urinary Ca+ excretion) • Ca+ supplements taken prior to blood draw	• Laxative use (increased intestinal Ca+ loss)

Related Tests:

Parathyroid hormone (PTH), thyroid panel, serum magnesium, RBC magnesium, serum phosphorous, serum albumin, total globulin, total protein, serum potassium, urinary calcium.

Serum Phosphorous

Background

The majority (85%) of the body's phosphorous is stored, in combination with calcium, in the bone. The remainder of the phosphorous is within the cells. Phosphorous in the blood exists as primarily inorganic phosphate in the form of HPO_4^{2-} or $H_2PO_4^-$, with the majority in the HPO_4^{2-} form, or as phosphate esters. It is difficult to determine the exact ratio between the two ionic forms of phosphorous, which is expressed as the total quantity of phosphorous.

Phosphorous is essential for bone matrix and hydroxyappetite metabolism. Phosphates play an important role in phospholipid and nucleic acid formation. It functions in the metabolism of glucose and lipids, is an important part of acid-base regulation and the storage and transfer of energy in the form of Adenosine Tri-Phosphate (ATP) and creatine phosphate.

Discussion

Phosphate levels are closely tied with calcium, but they are not as strictly controlled as calcium. Phosphorous levels, like calcium, are regulated by parathyroid hormone (PTH). Produced by the parathyroid gland, PTH is a very important hormone in phosphorous regulation. PTH promotes bone resorption of phosphorous, it has a very strong effect on the kidney causing excessive renal phosphate excretion, and enhances the absorption of phosphorous from the intestine through its effect on vitamin D. The net effect of PTH is to decrease serum phosphorous.

- On the cellular level, phosphate crosses the cell membrane with glucose. Plasma levels may be decreased after a high carbohydrate meal.

- Phosphorous levels should always be evaluated in relation to calcium because of the inverse relationship that exists between the two minerals. Phosphorous levels will be increased when calcium levels are decreased. When calcium levels increase, phosphorous levels will decrease. An excess in one of the minerals will cause an increase in renal excretion of the other.

- Serum phosphorous is a general marker for digestion. Decreased phosphorous levels are associated with hypochlorhydria.

- Phosphorous is often assumed to be a calcium antagonist. This may be true in its supplemental form but organic phosphorous from whole and unrefined foods is naturally buffered with minerals and vitamins that act as synergistic co-factors to increase calcium metabolism.

Common subjective indications of phosphorous need are:

1. Joint stiffness upon arising
2. Cold hands and feet
3. Joint soreness/stiffness after inactivity (sitting for over 30 minutes) that is improved with movement.

Ranges:

	Standard U.S. Units	Standard International Units
Conventional Laboratory Range	2.5 – 4.5 mg/dL	0.81 – 1.45 mmol/L
Optimal Range	3.0 – 4.0 mg/dL	0.97 – 1.29 mmol/L
Alarm Ranges	< 2.0 or > 5.0 mg/dL	< 0.65 or > 1.61 mmol/L

When would you run this test?

1. To ascertain digestive sufficiency

2. To monitor parathyroid function

Clinical implications

HIGH

Clinical Implication	Additional information
Parathyroid Hypofunction	Parathyroid hypofunction will lead to decreased PTH levels that can cause increase serum phosphorous.
	Pattern:
	If phosphorous is increased (>4.0 or 1.29 mmol/L) along with decreased calcium (<9.2 or 2.3 mmol/L), parathyroid hypofunction is **possible**. Alkaline phosphatase levels may also be normal or decreased (<70).

	Follow up with a serum parathyroid hormone test. If parathyroid hormone levels are also decreased presume clinical hypoparathyroidism exists.
Bone Growth (Children) And Bone Repair (Fractures)	An increased phosphorous (>4.0 or 1.29 mmol/L) is a normal finding in times of increased bone growth and bone repair. Serum phosphorous will often be > 5.0 with children up to 18 years of age (bone growth). Similar increases may be seen during bone repair (fractures).
Diet- excessive phosphate consumption	Serum phosphorous levels may be increased (>4.0 or 1.29 mmol/L) in people who drink a lot of soda pop. Phosphoric acid is a common additive in sodas and can lead to excessive levels of ingested phosphorous that can cause significant problems with the calcium/phosphorous ratio, leading to decreased serum calcium.
Renal Insufficiency	An increased phosphorous level can be a sign of renal insufficiency. Renal insufficiency is an often over-looked condition. **Please see the special topic on page 40 for more details.** **Pattern:** Suspect renal insufficiency if there is an increased serum phosphorous (>4.0 or 1.29 mmol/L) , an increased BUN level (>16 or 5.71 mmol/L) with a normal or increased serum creatinine (>1.1 or 97.2μmol/dL) and a normal to increased uric acid (>5.9 or > 351 μmol/dL). LDH and SGOT/AST will usually be normal.
Other conditions associated with increased phosphorous levels include	Edema · Renal dysfunction · Ovarian hyperfunction · Excess intake of vitamin D · Sarcoidosis · Bone Neoplasm · Diabetes · Liver dysfunction · Portal Cirrhosis · Excessive intake of antacids

LOW

Clinical Implication	Additional information
Parathyroid Hyperfunction	Parathyroid hyperfunction will cause an increase in PTH levels, which can lead to a decreased serum phosphorous.
	Pattern:
	If the serum phosphorous is decreased (<3.0 or <0.97 mmol/L) and the calcium is significantly increased (>10.5 or 2.63 mmol/L) parathyroid hyperfunction is **possible**. Alkaline phosphatase levels may also be increased (>100), along with a normal or decreased serum or RBC magnesium.
	Follow up with a serum parathyroid hormone test. If parathyroid hormone levels are also increased presume clinical hyperparathyroidism exists.
	✳ Hyperparathyroidism may be due to space-occupying lesions on one or more of the glands. Surgical removal may be necessary to determine if there is a neoplasm.
	✳ A patient with increased serum calcium and an increased PTH should be checked by an endocrinologist, as hyperparathyroidism is a serious condition.
Hypochlorhydria	A decreased serum phosphorous is associated with a decreased production of hydrochloric acid in the stomach (hypochlorhydria). **Please see the special topic on page 96 for more details on hypochlorhydria.**
	Pattern:
	🌰 Hypochlorhydria is **possible** with a decreased serum phosphorous (<3.0 or <0.97 mmol/L) and an increased or decreased globulin level (< 2.4 / 24 g/L or >2.8 / 28 g/L) and a normal or decreased total protein (<6.9 or 69 g/L).
	🌰 If the BUN is also increased (>16 or 5.71 mmol/L), hypochlorhydria is highly **probable**.
	Other values that may be reflective of a developing or chronic hypochlorhydria include increased or decreased gastrin (<50 or >100), an increased MCV (>90) and MCH (>31.9), a decreased or normal calcium (<9.2 or 2.3 mmol/L) and iron (< 50 or 8.96 μmol/dL), a decreased chloride (<100), an increased anion gap (>12) and a decreased alkaline phosphatase (<70).
	Some of clinical indications of hypochlorhydria include:
	1. Gas and bloating shortly after meals
	2. Sense of fullness/ easy satiety

	3. Nausea after taking supplements
	4. Weak, peeling, or cracked nails
	5. Dilated capillaries in cheeks and nose in non-alcoholics
Hyperinsulinism	Phosphate crosses the cell membrane with glucose. Hyperinsulinism, therefore, will cause an increased uptake of glucose by the cells and will also increase phosphorous uptake, possibly contributing to a decreased serum phosphorous level (<3.0 or 0.97 mmol/L).
Diet- high in refined carbohydrates	Phosphate crosses the cell membrane with glucose. Plasma levels may be decreased after a meal high in refined carbohydrates. A diet high in refined carbohydrates and sugars will deplete phosphorous stores and other important co-factors for carbohydrate metabolism.
Other conditions associated with decreased phosphorous levels include	Ovarian hypofunction Diabetes Vitamin D anemia Liver dysfunction Protein malnutrition

Interfering Factors:

Phosphorous has a diurnal rhythm, with higher levels noted in the afternoon or evening, which may be as much as double in the morning. Also has slight seasonal variation: highest in May and June, lowest in winter.

Falsely increased levels	Falsely decreased levels
• Laxatives or enemas containing sodium phosphate • Hemolysis of blood- separate serum from cells as soon as possible	• After a high carbohydrate meal- phosphorous enters the cell with glucose- can cause decreased serum levels

Related Tests:

Parathyroid hormone (PTH), thyroid panel, serum magnesium, RBC magnesium, serum calcium, serum albumin, total globulin, total protein, serum potassium, urinary calcium.

Serum Magnesium

Background

Magnesium is the second most common intracellular cation, after potassium. Only about 1-5% is found extracellularly. About half of the body's magnesium is found in the soft tissue and muscle cells. The remainder is found in the bone. About 1/3rd of dietary magnesium is absorbed. Absorption takes place in the small intestine.

Serum magnesium exists in three different forms in the plasma:

1. About 50% of the magnesium in the plasma is in the free/ionized form and is freely diffusible through the cell membrane.

2. 35% of the magnesium in the plasma is protein bound. Protein bound magnesium is primarily bound to albumin (75%) and globulins (25%).

3. The remaining 15% of the magnesium in the plasma is complexed to other substances, such as phosphate or citrate, and is freely diffusible through the cell membrane.

Magnesium is excreted by the kidney. Normally 95% of magnesium filtered by the glomerulus is reabsorbed in the tubule. Parathyroid hormone plays a role in regulating blood magnesium levels through its action on renal tubular reabsorption.

Magnesium is important for many different enzymatic reactions, including carbohydrate metabolism, protein synthesis, nucleic acid synthesis, and muscular contraction. Magnesium is also needed for oxidative phosphrylation and ATP production and is used by the body in the blood clotting mechanism.

Discussion

Serum magnesium is found intracellularly, and is therefore not the best method for assessing magnesium. If you need a more accurate assessment of magnesium, we recommend running a RED blood cell magnesium, because the RBCs contain 2-3 times the concentration of magnesium found in the serum. Refer to specific laboratory ranges when running an RBC level.

- Magnesium is closely associated with calcium. A deficiency of one can affect the metabolism of the other. Magnesium plays an important role in calcium absorption from the intestines. A magnesium deficiency causes calcium resorption from the bone, which may cause calcification

- Note: Part of the serum magnesium, like calcium, is bound to albumin. Check the serum albumin level to make sure that a decrease in serum albumin is not the cause for a relative serum magnesium decrease and an albumin increase is not the cause of a serum magnesium increase.

Common subjective indications of magnesium need are:

1. Muscle cramps
2. Chocolate craving
3. Chronic constipation
4. Dysrhythmia

Ranges:

	Standard U.S. Units	Standard International Units
Conventional Laboratory Range	1.5 – 2.3 mg/dL	0.62 – 0.95 mmol/L
Optimal Range	> 2.0 mg/dL	> 0.82 mmol/L
Alarm Ranges	< 1.2 mg/dL	< 0.49 mmol/L

When would you run this test?

1. Magnesium measurement is used as an index for metabolic activity.
2. Magnesium levels are measured to evaluate renal function and electrolytes status.

Clinical implications

HIGH

Clinical Implication	Additional information
Renal Dysfunction	Any type of kidney dysfunction (i.e. renal failure, infection, and blockage) can decrease kidney function, which causes increase magnesium retention, leading to increased serum

	levels of magnesium.
	Pattern:
	Increased BUN (>25 or 8.93 mmol/L), serum creatinine (>1.4 or 123.8 µmol/dL), BUN/Creatinine ratio (10-20), Urine specific gravity (1.010 - 1.016), Uric acid (>5.9 or > 351 µmol/dL), serum phosphorous (>4.0 or 1.29 mmol/L), LDH (>200), and SGOT/AST (>30). You may also see serum electrolytes outside of their metabolic range.
Thyroid hypofunction	Serum magnesium may be increased in either primary thyroid hypofunction or secondary thyroid hypofunction due to anterior pituitary hypofunction. Pattern: With primary hypothyroidism the magnesium levels may be increased along with a TSH increased (>4.0) With secondary thyroid hypofunction due to anterior pituitary hypofunction the magnesium levels may be increased along with a decreased TSH (<2.0)
Other conditions associated with increased magnesium levels include	Excessive Mg containing Antacids Dehydration Addison's disease

LOW

Clinical Implication	Additional information
Epilepsy	Decreased serum magnesium has been associated with epilepsy. Identifying an underlying magnesium need in people with epilepsy can be helpful. Some of the other considerations to think about in patients with epilepsy include: 1. Heavy metal body burden 2. Intestinal parasites 3. Hypoglycemia and blood sugar dysregulation 4. Liver dysfunction/toxicity 5. B6 deficiency **Pattern:** If serum magnesium levels are decreased along with a decreased SGOT/AST (<10), MCH (<28) and MCV (<82), magnesium and B6 should be considered as supportive agents

Muscle Spasm	The laboratory results with muscle spasm are variable; however, decreased serum or RBC magnesium is a common finding.
Other conditions associated with decreased magnesium levels include	Adrenal hyper-function Liver dysfunction Digestive inflammation Malabsorption Inflammation Hepatitis, Cirrhosis Chronic alcoholism Parathyroid hyperfunction Renal dysfunction (chronic renal disease)

Interfering Factors:

Falsely increased levels	Falsely decreased levels
• Aspirin use (prolonged) • Lithium therapy (Rx) • Magnesium products (Laxatives, Antacids) • Hemolytic problems (releases intracellular Magnesium) • Dehydration	• Calcium gluconate use (within 24 hrs of testing) • Hemodilution

Related Tests:

Serum calcium, parathyroid hormone (PTH), thyroid panel, serum phosphorous, serum albumin, total globulin, total protein, serum potassium, urinary calcium, CO_2 and anion gap. With fibromyalgia, CO_2 will frequently be decreased, with an increased anion gap and a decreased serum or RBC magnesium.

Alkaline Phosphatase

Background

Alkaline phosphatase (ALP) is a group of isoenzymes that originate in the bone, liver, intestines, skin, and placenta. It has a maximal activity at a pH of 9.0-10.0, hence the term alkaline phosphatase. ALP is a member of the metaloprotein family of enzymes that remove phosphate from organic phosphate esters. Metaloenzymes are zinc dependent for their optimal function, and decreased levels of ALP have been associated with zinc deficiency. The total ALP level is composed of fractions of ALP isoenzymes. Each of these isoenzymes can be fractionated by electrophoresis into their constituent fraction.

Discussion

 In the liver, ALP is formed by liver and biliary mucosal cells, and is excreted in the bile by a mechanism that is different than bilirubin excretion. Elevated levels in the serum can occur with any liver dysfunction, it is especially sensitive to **any type** of obstruction in the biliary tract, both intra and extra-hepatic, both severe and mild. The degree of ALP elevation is in direct correlation to the severity of the obstruction.

- The most common liver causes of increased serum ALP include extra-hepatic or common bile duct obstruction, intra-hepatic biliary tract obstruction that is usually caused by acute damage to the liver cells (viral hepatitis, active cirrhosis), and space-occupying tumors in the liver, especially metastatic tumors of the liver. Mild elevations of ALP may be seen in patients with fatty liver.

 Elevations of ALP have been associated with drug-induced liver damage and are a sign that a drug toxicity reaction is occurring.

- ALP of bone origin is the most common extra-hepatic source of increased ALP levels. Large amounts of ALP are produced by osteoblastic activity in the bone, which is usually seen in normal bone growth in children and healing fractures. Abnormal elevations are seen in diseases of the bone that have hyperactivity in osteoblastic activity and in metastatic carcinoma from a number of different organs that metastasize to the bone.

119

ALP and Blood Type/Secretor Status

There is some evidence to suggest that different blood types and secretor status will have an impact on normal ALP levels. For instance, people with O and B blood groups, especially those that are Lewis positive secretors, will have an elevated ALP, especially of intestinal origin, 2-4 hours after a fatty meal.

Intestinal ALP is involved in the breakdown of dietary cholesterol and calcium absorption. People with type O blood tend to have the highest intestinal ALP activity. People with type A blood tend to have the lowest intestinal ALP activity. This may help explain why people with O type blood are better equipped to deal with cholesterol-containing foods (meats etc.) and why people with type A blood, with the lowest amounts of intestinal ALP, have great difficulty dealing with dietary fat and cholesterol containing foods.

- Any patient who has a significantly elevated total serum ALP should be followed up with an ALP isoenzyme study, which will help pinpoint the tissue involved in the total serum ALP increase.

Ranges:

	Standard U.S. Units	Standard International Units
Conventional Laboratory Range	25 – 120 U/L	25 – 120 U/L
Optimal Range	70 – 100 U/L	70 – 100 U/L
Alarm Ranges	<30 U/L or > 130 U/L	<30 U/L or > 130 U/L

When would you run this test?

1. Evaluating liver dysfunction
2. To monitor the severity of biliary dysfunction
3. Evaluating bone disorders
4. Alkaline phosphatase, along with the associated isoenzymes, is used as a tumor marker

Clinical implications

HIGH

Clinical Implication	Additional information
Biliary Obstruction	Alkaline phosphatase levels rise when excretion is blocked by an obstruction somewhere in the biliary tree. Increased alkaline phosphatase (>100) along with an increased GGTP (>30) is seen with biliary tree involvement. If the problem involves a biliary/common bile duct obstruction, the alkaline phosphatase and the GGTP will generally be increased significantly above the SGPT/ALT. If there is an actual stone or calculi the total bilirubin level will also be elevated (>1.2 or 20.5µmol/dL). Suspect biliary involvement if there are strong subjective and a history of the following indicators: 1. Nausea 2. Gallbladder attacks (past or present) 3. Headache over the eye 4. Bitter taste in the mouth 5. Greasy or high fat foods cause distress 6. Pain between shoulder blades 7. Light brown or yellow stools
Liver cell damage	If alkaline phosphatase levels are increased (>100) with increased total bilirubin (>1.2 or 20.5 µmol/dL), direct bilirubin (>0.2 or 3.4 µmol/dL), SGOT/AST (>30), GGTP (>30), and/or LDH (>200) liver dysfunction is **probable**. This may be caused by cellular damage, such as liver infection (hepatitis, infectious mononucleosis, EBV, CMV, etc.), which should be ruled out. An increase in ALP can be an indicator of liver dysfunction due to drug toxicities. Ask you patients about their prescription and non-prescription drug use. Elevated levels of ALP are often seen in patients with metastatic carcinoma of the liver, which will cause an increase in the liver fraction of ALP.
Bone loss or increased bone turnover due to: • **Osteomalacia** • **Rickets**	In bone disease, the alkaline phosphatase enzyme levels rise in proportion to new bone cell production. This results from both an increased calcium deposition in the bones and increased osteoblastic activity. Alkaline phosphatase can be used to differentiate osteomalacia from osteoporosis, in which there is no apparent elevation. Osteoporosis and/or osteomalacia can be confirmed with radiological studies,

• **Paget's disease** • **Rheumatoid arthritis** • **Hodgkin's lymphoma**	which will show bone loss, and urinary hydroxyproline excretion, which increases as the alkaline phosphatase bone isoenzyme increases and the bone loss becomes more severe. Bone loss can also be assessed with densiometry studies. The alkaline phosphatase isoenzyme that corresponds to the bone will be elevated. It is important in these situations to assess the bone loss and support the condition with appropriate mineral support.
Bone growth and repair- fracture healing	Alkaline phosphatase enzyme levels will often be increased in situations of bone growth and repair. Increased osteoblastic activity, along with calcium deposition in the bones will cause this increase.
"Leaky Gut" syndrome	Alkaline phosphatase can have an intestinal origin. The intestinal ALP is involved with dietary cholesterol breakdown and calcium absorption. Increased levels are often seen in conditions involving the intestinal mucosa e.g. leaky gut syndrome, ulcers, colitis, and malabsorption. Serum gastrin levels may also be elevated. Many organisms (bacteria, yeast, amoebas) and their toxins are easily absorbed in a compromised digestive barrier, setting up a resultant auto-immune response in many cases. Treatment should be oriented to restoring gut integrity and correcting the dysbiotic terrain. Note that a reaction is common initially (Herxheimer reaction) as an increased release of endotoxins occurs during early treatment.
Herpes Zoster (shingles)	Although best determined from a physical examination of the lesions, shingles will often result in an elevated ALP. With the inflammation of shingles, the sedimentation rate, C-reactive protein, and basophil count will often be increased, while the total WBC levels, viral titers and SGPT/ALT will often be normal.
Metastatic carcinoma of the bone	Due to the elevated bone destruction and attempts by the body to repair, elevated levels of ALP significantly above the reference range can occur in metastatic carcinoma of the bone from carcinomas of the prostate (70-90% of patients), breast (50% of patients), and about 30% of patients with metastatic carcinoma of the lung, kidney or thyroid.
Vitamin C need	An increased Alkaline phosphatase level is associated with vitamin C need. **Pattern:** 🍁 Albumin will frequently be decreased (<4.0 or 40g/L) along a decreased HCT (<37 or 0.37 in women and 40 or 0.4 in

	men), HGB (<13.5 or 135 g/L in women and <14 or 140 men), MCH (<28), MCHC (<32), serum iron (< 50 or 8.96 μmol/dL). There will also be an increased MCV (>90), alkaline phosphatase (>100), and fibrinogen. Both the lingual ascorbic acid test and Urinary vitamin C will generally be out of range. **Please see the special topic on the lingual ascorbic acid test on page 218 for more details.**	
Other conditions associated with increased ALP levels include	Excess ingestion of vitamin D Excessive fat and/or protein intake Adrenal hyperfunction Renal dysfunction Pancreatic dysfunction	Tissue damage Hyperthyroidism Alcoholism Liver cirrhosis Hepatitis Infectious mononucleosis Cancer

LOW

Clinical Implication	Additional information
Zinc deficiency 	Alkaline phosphatase is a zinc dependent enzyme. Decreased levels (<70) have been associated with zinc deficiency along with decreased WBC or RBC zinc levels and a low normal or decreased total WBC. Follow up an increased alkaline phosphatase with a zinc taste test. Some of the clinical signs of zinc deficiency include: 1. White spots on nails 2. Reduced sense of smell or taste 3. Cuts are slow to heal 4. Acne 5. Susceptible to colds, infections, and flu 6. BPH

Zinc Taste Test

The zinc taste test is a non-invasive method of determining a patient's physiological zinc status. The patient holds a small amount of a 0.1% zinc sulfate solution in their mouth for 15 seconds to assess their ability to taste the solution. Optimal zinc levels are seen in patients that have an immediate and unpleasant taste in their mouth. Zinc insufficiency is seen in patients for whom the solution has no apparent taste. When the Alkaline phosphatase is below 70 U/L and the above subjective indications for deficiency are present, treat for zinc deficiency with 100mg of zinc/day for 30 days

Drug causes of ↓	✲ Estrogen ✲ Estrogen in combination with androgens	
Other conditions associated with decreased ALP levels include	⬤ Hypothyroidism ⬤ Very low fat and low protein diets	⬤ Adrenal hypofunction ✲ Pernicious anemia

Interfering Factors:

Falsely increased levels	Falsely decreased levels
• Pregnancy, especially the 3rd trimester • Young children experiencing rapid growth • Phenytoin	• Anticoagulated blood sample

Related Tests:

Isoenzymes of ALP, LDH, and LDH isoenzymes, total bilirubin, SGOT/AST, SGPT/ALT, GGTP, Serum protein electrophoresis, total protein, serum albumin, serum globulin, WBC and differential, thyroid panel, serum calcium and phosphorous

Alkaline Phosphatase Isoenzymes

Discussion

The total alkaline phosphatase level is composed of fractions of 6 ALP isoenzymes. Each of these isoenzymes can be fractionated by electrophoresis into their constituent fraction. Anyone with a significantly increased total ALP level should have an ALP isoenzyme study performed. An increase in one or more of the isoenzymes is indicative of a problem in the specific tissue that correlates with the elevated isoenzymes.

Isoenzyme	Background
Liver Isoenzyme a2	• Major ALP isoenzyme in the liver. • Most frequently increased with an increased total serum ALP. • Increases seen in early liver disease. May even be increased before other liver function tests are positive.
Liver Isoenzyme a1	• Isoenzyme a1 is known as the "fast liver isoenzyme". • Strongly associated with metastatic liver cancer
Bone Isoenzyme	• Increased levels of osteoblastic activity in the bone will contribute to increased ALP bone isoenzyme levels. • Will be increased with normal bone growth and healing of fractures.
Intestinal Isoenzyme	• People with O and B blood groups, especially those that are Lewis positive secretors, will have an elevated intestinal ALP isoenzyme 2-4 hours after a fatty meal. Intestinal ALP is involved in the breakdown of dietary cholesterol and calcium absorption. • Associated with ulcerative or erosive lesions. • People with type O blood have the highest .intestinal ALP activity. • People with type A blood have the lowest intestinal ALP activity.

***Placental* Isoenzyme**	• This fraction is normally increased in pregnancy and can cause an elevated total serum ALP in pregnancy.
***Regan* or Regan variant**	• The fraction associated with several types of cancer.

Ranges:

	Isoenzyme	Conventional Laboratory range:
Standard U.S. Units	Liver Isoenzyme a2 Liver Isoenzyme a1 Bone Isoenzyme Intestinal Isoenzyme Placental Isoenzyme Regan or regan variant	All values are reported as weak, moderate or strong

When would you run this test?

1. ALP Isoenzymes are excellent for differentiating benign from cancerous liver conditions

2. Can be used to identify liver, bone, and intestinal conditions and diseases with or without an increase in total serum ALP.

Conditions associated with elevated ALP isoenzymes

Isoenzyme	Conditions
Liver Isoenzyme a2	✺ Hepatitis ✺ Cirrhosis ◉ Fatty liver ✺ Drug induced liver disease ◉ Biliary obstruction ✺ Liver cancer
Liver Isoenzyme a1	✺ Metastatic liver cancer ✺ Viral hepatitis ✺ Cirrhosis- especially alcohol induced along with ↑ GGTP, should be ruled out

Bone Isoenzyme	<ul><li>Paget's disease</li><li>Rickets</li><li>Bone cancer</li><li>Osteomalacia</li><li>Osteoporosis</li><li>Primary parathyroid hyperfunction</li><li>Urinary hydroxyproline excretion increases as the ALP bone isoenzyme increases especially with osteoporosis, osteomalacia, and parathyroid hyperfunction</li></ul>
Intestinal Isoenzyme	<ul><li>Perforated bowel</li><li>Ulcerative diseases of intestinal mucosa in stomach, duodenum, small intestine, and colon</li><li>Lesions associated with malabsorption if there is erosion or ulceration</li></ul>
Placental Isoenzyme	<ul><li>Normally elevated in pregnancy</li><li>May become significantly increased in toxemia of pregnancy that can cause infarction of the placenta</li></ul>
Regan or Regan variant	<ul><li>Lung cancer</li><li>Colon cancer</li><li>Ovarian cancer</li><li>Hepatocellular cancer</li><li>Pancreatic cancer</li></ul>

Interfering Factors:

Falsely increased levels	Falsely decreased levels
<ul><li>Pregnancy, especially the 3rd trimester</li><li>Young children experiencing rapid growth</li><li>Phenytoin</li></ul>	<ul><li>Anticoagulated blood sample</li></ul>

Related Tests:

Total serum ALP, LDH and LDH isoenzymes, total bilirubin, SGOT/AST, SGPT/ALT, GGTP, Serum protein electrophoresis, total protein, serum albumin, serum globulin, WBC and differential, thyroid panel, serum calcium, and phosphorous

SGOT/AST

Background

SGOT/AST is an enzyme present in highly metabolic tissues such as skeletal muscle, the liver, the heart, kidney, and lungs. This enzyme is at times liberated into the bloodstream following cell damage or destruction.

Aspartate aminotransferase, or AST or SGOT, is the enzyme that catalyzes the conversion of the amino acid L-aspartate and α-keto-glutarate into oxaloacetate and L-glutamate, hence the older name SGOT or Serum Glutamate-Oxaloacetate Transaminase.

Discussion

SGOT/AST is functionally similar to SGPT/ALT, however in liver problems it is not as increased as SGPT/ALT. SGOT/AST is more specific for the detection of problems of cardiovascular origin than for biliary tree or liver problems. Levels originating from the liver are due to damage to the hepatocytes or liver cells.

- AST levels will be increased when liver cells and/or heart muscle cells and/or skeletal muscle cells are damaged. The cause of the damage must be investigated.

- AST levels in the blood due to severe cellular damage will usually increase in 12 hours and remain elevated for about 5 days.

- In acute episodes the AST levels will return to normal in 3-6 days.

Ranges:

	Standard U.S. Units	Standard International Units
Conventional Laboratory Range	0 – 40 U/L	0 – 40 U/L
Optimal Range	10 – 30 U/L	10 – 30 U/L
Alarm Ranges	> 100 U/L	> 100 U/L

When would you run this test?

1. To investigate cardiovascular and/or liver problems
2. As a gateway test for B6 deficiency

Clinical implications

HIGH

Clinical Implication	Additional information
Dysfunction located outside the liver and biliary tree	If the SGOT/AST is increased above the levels of the SGPT/ALT and GGTP consider that the problem or area of involvement is possible outside the liver and biliary tree (i.e. the heart, gall bladder, common bile duct, and pancreas)
A developing Congestive heart picture	An increased SGOT/AST level (>30) can be an important clue to this very common cardiovascular disease. Other indicators may include: 1. Poor oxygenation/air hunger or yawn frequently 2. Shortness of breath with moderate exertion 3. Edema/ankles swell, especially at end of the day 4. Cough when prostrate, especially at night **Pattern:** If SGOT/AST is increased higher than an accompanying SGPT/ALT increase with a normal to increased GGTP (>30), increased alkaline phosphatase (>100) and a decreased CO_2 (<25) consider the possibility of a developing congestive heart failure. It is more likely with an increased ESR, normal to increased globulin (>and LDH, and an increased uric acid (>5.9 or 351 μmol/dL).
Cardiovascular dysfunction: Coronary artery insufficiency	An increase in this enzyme can be suggestive of atherosclerotic changes in the coronary vasculature. Other indicators may include: 1. Reduced circulation/cold hands and feet 2. Angina/Muscle cramps with exertion 3. Blush or face turns red with no apparent reason **Pattern:** If SGOT/AST is increased higher than an accompanying SGPT/ALT increase with an increased CO_2 and uric acid, consider the possibility of coronary artery insufficiency, especially if RBC magnesium is decreased.

Acute Myocardial Infarct	With a suspected or an acute MI, the SGOT/AST is increased 4-10 times above the reference range, peaking after 24 hours and normalizing after 3-4 days. Secondary rises in SGOT/AST levels suggest a recurring MI or continued infarction.

Differentiating Cardiovascular Risk Profiles

The cardiovascular profile can be significantly different in individuals depending on multiple metabolic factors. Those with a predisposition to a longer-term degenerative cardiovascular picture constitute the "CHF" type. Whereas, the "MI" type will often have very few clinical indicators that tend to be well masked by compensatory mechanisms.

"MI" Type	"CHF" Type
• Hypertensive/vascular hypertonicity	• Hypotensive/poor vascular tone
• Craves alcohol	• Craves sugar
• Feels good/ pumped	• Feels Bad/Run down
• Doesn't get sick	• Sick often
• Muscular spasms	• Tend to be acidotic with shortness of breath
• Especially those with **adrenal** problems	• Especially those with **thyroid** problems
• Lack B2 (riboflavin)	• Lack B1 (Thiamine)
• Problems with Fat metabolism	• Problems with Carbohydrate metabolism

Liver cell damage	Liver damage due to active cellular destruction (i.e. chronic/acute hepatitis, active cirrhosis, infectious mononucleosis, hepatic necrosis, alcoholic hepatitis) will usually result in SGOT/AST values 10-100 times above reference range.
Liver dysfunction	An increased SGOT/AST (>30) is associated with liver dysfunction. Dysfunction in the liver may cause an increase in SGOT/AST from hepatocytes. Functionally oriented liver problems, such as detoxification issues, liver congestion, and conjugation problems are extremely common and should be evaluated based upon early prognostic indicators. The liver should always be viewed in the context of the hepato-biliary tree. Some of the key clinical

	indicators include: 1. Pain between shoulder blades 2. Stomach upset by greasy foods 3. If drinking alcohol, easily intoxicated 4. Headache over the eye 5. Sensitive to chemicals (perfume, cleaning solvents, insecticides, exhaust, etc.) 6. Hemorrhoids or varicose veins
Excessive muscle breakdown or turnover	SGOT/AST is present in high concentrations in tissues with high metabolic activity, such as skeletal muscle. Conditions or situations that cause cellular damage to skeletal muscle cells may cause an increased SGOT/AST level (i.e. weight training injuries, trauma to skeletal muscle, polymyositis)
Infectious mononucleosis, Epstein Barr and Cytomegalovirus	SGOT/AST levels are usually elevated way above the normal reference level about 5-14 days after the onset of illness. Alkaline phosphatase levels will also be elevated. LDH levels are usually elevated in about 95% of cases of. You may expect the following changes: ↓ WBCs in first week, ↑ WBCs by 2nd week of illness, ↑ GGTP (about 7-21 days after onset of illness).
Other conditions associated with increased SGOT/AST levels include	Free radical pathology Metastatic cancer Biliary dysfunction Acute and chronic pancreatitis Asthma Alcoholism

LOW

Clinical Implication	Additional information
B6 Deficiency	Vitamin B6, in its active form of pyridoxyl-5-phosphate (P-5-P), is essential for the effective operation of the transferase enzymes. A deficiency in P-5-P from alcoholism, malnutrition, poor assimilation, deficiencies in the diet, etc. will cause decreased levels of aminotransferase enzymes, such as SGOT/AST in general circulation. **Pattern:** B6 deficiency is likely if there is a decreased SGOT/AST (<10) and a concomitant deficiency in GGTP (<10) and/or SGPT/ALT (<10), enzymes that also need B6 for optimum activity. B6 deficiency can also impact red blood cell activity leading to a decreased MCV (<82) and/or MCH (<28) and a

	normal serum iron and ferritin level. This situation leads to a B6 deficiency anemia.
Alcoholism	Alcoholism is well known to deplete vitamin B6 from the body. Vitamin B6, in its active form of pyridoxyl-5-phosphate (P-5-P), is essential for the effective operation of the aminotransferase enzymes. A deficiency in P-5-P from alcoholism will cause decreased levels of SGOT/AST in general circulation.
Other conditions associated with decreased SGOT/AST levels include	Protein deficiency Malabsorption Gonadal hypofunction Kidney failure

Interfering Factors:

Falsely increased levels	Falsely decreased levels
• Salicylates and alcohol	• Slight decreases during **pregnancy** because of abnormal metabolism of pyridoxine • Salicylates and alcohol

Related Tests:

SGPT/ALT, GGTP, total serum bilirubin, serum ALP and ALP isoenzymes, serum LDH and LDH isoenzymes, total serum globulin, serum iron, serum ferritin, WBC and differential, EBV and CMV titers, hepatitis A, B, and C, mononucleosis, serum albumin, BUN, serum uric acid, serum and RBC magnesium

SGPT/ALT

Background

SGPT/ALT is an enzyme present in high concentrations in the liver and to lesser extent skeletal muscle, the heart, and kidney. SGPT/ALT will be liberated into the bloodstream following cell damage or destruction.

Alanine aminotransferase, or ALT or SGPT, is the enzyme that catalyzes the conversion of the amino acid L-alanine and α keto-glutarate into pyruvate and L-glutamate, hence the older name SGPT or Serum Glutamate-Pyruvate Transaminase.

Discussion

SGPT/ALT is functionally similar to SGOT/AST, however in liver problems it is increased more than SGOT/AST. SGPT/ALT is more specific for the detection of biliary tree or liver problems than problems of cardiovascular origin. Levels originating from the liver are due to damage to the hepatocytes or liver cells.

- Any condition or situation that causes damage to the hepatocytes will cause a leakage of SGPT/ALT in to the bloodstream.

- SGPT/ALT levels tend to take a long time to normalize after an elevation. This is in contrast to SGOT/AST levels, which will normalize quite quickly after an elevation. This can be used clinically to differentiate a chronic from an acute problem.

- SGPT/ALT levels, due to its concentration in the hepatocytes, are key in monitoring situations that can cause damage to the liver e.g. exposure to chemicals, viral hepatitis, alcoholic hepatitis

Ranges:

	Standard U.S. Units	Standard International Units
Conventional Laboratory Range	0 – 45 U/L	0 – 45 U/L
Optimal Range	10 – 30 U/L	10 – 30 U/L
Alarm Ranges	> 100 U/L	> 100 U/L

When would you run this test?

1. To determine whether or not damage to the liver has occurred

2. As part of a liver function panel

3. To help differentiate between hemolytic jaundice and jaundice caused by liver disease

Clinical implications

HIGH

Clinical Implication	Additional information
Dysfunction located inside the liver	If the SGPT/ALT is increased above the levels of the SGOT/AST and GGTP consider that the problem or area of involvement is **possibly** inside the liver
Fatty liver (steatosis)	Liver dysfunction due to fatty liver is possible when the SGPT/ALT levels are elevated within 4 times the upper limit of normal (<140), accompanied with an elevation in SGOT/AST. SGPT/ALT is usually greater then the SGPT/AST level. This is an opposite pattern to alcoholic hepatitis. GGTP may or may not be elevated, as it correlates with liver fat but it is not very sensitive to the presence of steatosis.
	Pattern:
	If the SGPT/ALT is increased (>30) above the SGOT/AST and GGTP levels (>30), liver dysfunction due to fatty liver is **probable**. Consider it more likely if the LDH (>200) and ALP levels (>100) are also increased.
Liver dysfunction	An increased SGPT/ALT (>30) is associated with liver dysfunction. Dysfunction in the liver may cause an increase in SGPT/ALT from hepatocytes.
	Functionally oriented liver problems, such as detoxification issues, liver congestion, and conjugation problems are extremely common and should be evaluated based upon early prognostic indicators. The liver should always be viewed in the context of the hepato-biliary tree. Some of the key clinical indicators include:
	1. Pain between shoulder blades
	2. Stomach upset by greasy foods
	3. If drinking alcohol, easily intoxicated

	4. Headache over the eye
	5. Sensitive to chemicals (perfume, cleaning solvents, insecticides, exhaust, etc.)
	6. Hemorrhoids or varicose veins
Biliary tract obstruction (due to liver dysfunction)	Conditions that cause damage to the liver cells (alcohol-induced injury, viral hepatitis, EBV, infectious mononucleosis, liver congestion, CMV) can cause obstruction in the small biliary channels between the liver cell groups that form the functional units of the liver and create a situation of liver dysfunction. SGPT/ALT levels will be elevated. Serum bilirubin levels will be elevated along with both conjugated and unconjugated fractions. The unconjugated fraction may be increased due to the liver's decreased ability to conjugate bilirubin due to liver cell damage.
	Pattern:
	Suspect biliary tract obstruction due to liver dysfunction when the SGPT/ALT is elevated (>30) with increased GGTP (>30), total bilirubin (>1.2 or >20.5 μmol/dL), alkaline phosphatase (>100) and/or LDH (>200).
	Liver infection: hepatitis, CMV, EBV, Infectious mononucleosis, etc. should be ruled out.
Excessive muscle breakdown or turnover	SGPT/ALT is an essential enzyme in the glucose-alanine cycle. Hard-working skeletal muscle functions anaerobically and produces large amounts of ammonia from protein breakdown and pyruvate from glycolysis. Alanine serves as the carrier of the ammonia and pyruvate from the hard-working skeletal muscle to the liver. In the liver the ammonia is converted into urea and the pyruvate is converted into glucose by gluconeogenesis and returned to the muscle.
	Conditions such as weight-training and muscular injury can cause elevated levels of ALT to appear in the bloodstream.
Cirrhosis of the liver	An increase SGPT/ALT is associated with liver cirrhosis
	Pattern:
	✳ Suspect liver cirrhosis if SGPT/ALT (>45) is increased along with an increased SGOT/AST (>40) and GGTP (>70), with a decreased serum albumin (<4.0 or 40g/L), increased serum ALP (>200), increased serum bilirubin (>1.2 or >20.5 μmol/dL), decreased cholesterol (<150 or 3.9 mmol/L), increased globulin (>2.8 or 28 g/L), increased LDH (>200)
	This pattern is generally seen with multiple types of cirrhosis –

	further clinical investigation is necessary to determine type and extent of problem (LDH isoenzymes, ALP isoenzyme a1 and a2, alpha 2 globulin)
Liver cell damage	Liver damage due to active cellular destruction (i.e. chronic/acute hepatitis, active cirrhosis, infectious mononucleosis, hepatic necrosis, alcoholic hepatitis) will usually result in significantly elevated SGPT/ALT values (30-50 times higher than normal)
Drug causes of ↑	❋ Salicylate poisoning

Other conditions associated with increased SGPT/ALT levels include	◉ Free radical pathology ◉ Biliary dysfunction ❋ Metastatic carcinoma	❋ Pancreatitis ❋ MI/ Ischemic heart disease ❋ Alcoholism

LOW

Clinical Implication	Additional information
B6 Deficiency	Vitamin B6, in its active form of pyridoxyl-5-phosphate (P-5-P), is essential for the effective operation of the transferase enzymes. A deficiency in P-5-P from alcoholism, malnutrition, poor assimilation, deficiencies in the diet, etc. will cause decreased levels of aminotransferase enzymes such as SGOT/AST in general circulation. **Pattern:** B6 deficiency is likely if there is a decreased SGOT/AST (<10) and a concomitant deficiency in GGTP (<10) and/or SGPT/ALT (<10), enzymes that also need B6 for optimum activity. B6 deficiency can also impact red blood cell activity leading to a decreased MCV/MCH and a normal serum iron and ferritin level. This situation leads to a B6 deficiency anemia.
Fatty liver (early development) **(Steatosis)**	A decreased SGPT/ALT (<10) is associated with liver congestion and the early development of fatty liver (steatosis). Fatty liver is caused by obesity, excessive alcohol consumption, prescription drugs (e.g. steroids), iron overload, solvent exposure, and rapid weight loss. Fatty changes to the liver tissue can lead to a decreased output of SGPT/AST from the hepatocytes. Fatty changes can also impair the liver's detoxification ability. The degree of fatty liver changes is

	directly related to the amount of obesity.
	Pattern:
	If total cholesterol (>220 or 5.69 mmol/L), LDL (>120 or 3.1 mmol/L), and triglyceride levels (>110 or 1.24 mmol/L) are increased, and HDL levels are decreased (<55 or 1.42 mmol/L), then the early development of fatty liver is **possible**.
Liver congestion	Liver congestion, due to the beginning stages of steatosis (fatty liver), should be considered if total cholesterol is above 220 or 5.69 mmol/L, triglycerides are increased (>110 or 1.24 mmol/L), and the SGPT/ALT is below 10. Fatty liver and liver congestion increase the risk of insulin resistance, hypertension, Metabolic Syndrome, and type II diabetes mellitus.
Alcoholism	Alcoholism is well known to deplete vitamin B6 from the body. Vitamin B6, in its active form of pyridoxyl-5-phosphate (P-5-P), is essential for the effective operation of the aminotransferase enzymes. A deficiency in P-5-P from alcoholism will cause decreased levels of SGPT/ALT (<10) in general circulation.
Other conditions associated with decreased SGPT/ALT levels include	Protein deficiency Kidney failure Malabsorption

Interfering Factors:

Falsely increased levels	Falsely decreased levels
• Salicylates	• Salicylates

Related Tests:

SGOT/AST, GGTP, total serum bilirubin, serum ALP and ALP isoenzymes, serum LDH and LDH isoenzymes, total serum globulin, serum iron, serum ferritin, WBC and differential, EBV and CMV titers, hepatitis A, B and C, mononucleosis, serum albumin, BUN, serum uric acid, serum and RBC magnesium

GGTP

Background

Gamma Glutamyl Transferase (GGTP) is an enzyme that is present in highest amounts in the liver cells and to a lesser extent the kidney, prostate, and pancreas. It is also found in the epithelial cells of the biliary tract. It is involved in amino acid and protein metabolism by transferring the C-terminal glutamic acid from a peptide to other peptides or amino acids. GGTP will be liberated into the bloodstream following cell damage or destruction and/or biliary obstruction.

Discussion

GGTP is a much more sensitive and specific marker for hepatic dysfunction than serum ALP and SGPT/ALT for some conditions (cholangitis, cholecystitis, obstructive jaundice). GGTP is generally increased above the other liver enzymes with biliary tree problems (gall bladder, common bile duct, and pancreas), obstruction, or alcoholism.

- GGTP levels may be elevated by as high as 50% in patients with obesity.

- GGTP is induced by alcohol and can be elevated following chronic alcohol consumption and in alcoholism. It is therefore used as a screen for the consequences of chronic alcoholism and to detect alcohol induced liver disease. GGTP levels are normally not affected by a moderate alcohol intake.

- Men may present with high normal levels due to the large amounts of GGTP found in the prostate

Ranges:

	Standard U.S. Units	Standard International Units
Conventional Laboratory Range	1 – 70 U/L	1 – 70 U/L
Optimal Range	10 – 30 U/L	10 – 30 U/L
Alarm Ranges	> 90 U/L	> 90 U/L

When would you run this test?

1. To identify biliary tree problems (gallbladder, common bile duct, pancreas)
2. To identify obstructive disease of the bile tract
3. To identify and/or monitor alcoholism

Clinical implications

HIGH

Clinical Implication	Additional information
Dysfunction located outside the liver and inside the biliary tree	If the GGTP is increased above the levels of the SGPT/ALT and SGOT/AST consider that the problem or area of involvement is possible outside the liver but inside the biliary tree (i.e. gall bladder, common bile duct, and pancreas)
Biliary obstruction	GGTP levels rise when excretion is blocked by an obstruction somewhere in the biliary tree. Increased GGTP along with an increased alkaline phosphatase is seen with biliary tree involvement. There will usually be significant increases in GGTP (greater than 5 times higher than normal). **Pattern:** If GGTP (>30) and alkaline phosphatase (>100) are increased along with a normal or increased SGOT/AST (>30) and SGPT/ALT (>30), biliary obstruction with possible calculi is **probable**. Biliary obstruction with possible calculi becomes even more likely with an increased total bilirubin (>1.2 or 20.5 µmol/dL) and direct bilirubin (>0.2 or 3.4 µmol/dL).
Biliary stasis or insufficiency	Biliary stasis or insufficiency can often be caused by a mild obstruction in the extra-hepatic biliary duct. GGTP levels will frequently be increased (>30) but not necessarily. Bilirubin levels will also be elevated (>1.2 or 20.5 µmol/dL) along with alkaline phosphatase (>100) and total cholesterol (>220 or 5.69 mmol/L). SGOT/AST and SGPT/ALT may be normal or increased (>30). Many cases of biliary stasis will show normal lab values. In these situations suspect biliary stasis or insufficiency if there are strong subjective indicators: 1. Pain between shoulder blades 2. Stomach upset by greasy foods 3. Greasy or shiny stools 4. Nausea 5. Light or clay colored stools 6. Gallbladder attacks 7. Headache over the eye 8. Bitter taste in mouth, especially after meals
Liver cell damage	Another common cause of an increased GGTP level is active or acute liver cell damage (i.e. chronic/acute hepatitis, active cirrhosis, infectious mononucleosis, hepatic necrosis,

	alcoholic hepatitis). There will usually be moderate increases in GGTP 3-5 times higher than normal (200 - 300).
Excessive alcohol consumption, alcoholism	Increased GGTP without an increase in the other liver enzymes suggests excessive alcohol consumption. If GGTP is increased (>30) along with an increased serum triglyceride level (>110 or 1.24 mmol/L), excess alcohol use should be ruled out. Excessive alcohol use can seriously affect the liver function, therefore we may also see elevated SGOT/AST (>30) and SGPT/ALT levels (>30), but the GGTP will usually be higher.
Acute or chronic pancreatitis	Suspect pancreatic pathology if the GGTP is increased 5 times higher than the normal i.e. 320 U/L or higher
Pancreatic insufficiency	Mild to moderate chronic pancreatitis can lead to a pancreatic insufficiency over time. In these cases GGTP levels may be mild to moderately increased (>30). One of the most significant contributing factors to pancreatic insufficiency is an accompanying hypochlorhydria picture. Some of the clinical implications of pancreatic insufficiency include: 1. Undigested food in the stool 2. Food allergies 3. Indigestion 4. Diarrhea 5. Sense of excess fullness after meals 6. Sleepy after meals especially one high in carbohydrates

Other conditions associated with increased GGTP levels include	Free radical pathology Parasites Hyperthyroidism Congestive heart failure	Diabetes Asthma Liver metastasis and carcinoma

LOW

Clinical Implication	Additional information
B6 Deficiency	Vitamin B6, in its active form of pyridoxyl-5-phosphate (P-5-P), is essential for the effective operation of the transferase enzymes. A deficiency in P-5-P from alcoholism, malnutrition, poor assimilation, deficiencies in the diet, etc. will cause decreased levels of aminotransferase enzymes, such as SGOT/AST in general circulation.

	Pattern: B6 deficiency is likely if there is a decreased SGOT/AST (<10) and a concomitant deficiency in GGTP (<10) and/or SGPT/ALT (<10), enzymes that also need B6 for optimum activity. B6 deficiency can also impact red blood cell activity leading to a decreased MCV (<82) and/or MCH (<82) and a normal serum iron and ferritin level. This situation leads to a B6 deficiency anemia.
Magnesium need	A low GGTP (<10) is associated with a need for magnesium. Magnesium levels can be assessed using RBC or WBC magnesium levels. Some of the clinical signs of a potential magnesium deficiency are: 1. Muscle cramps 2. Chocolate craving 3. Chronic constipation 4. Dysrhythmia
Other conditions associated with decreased GGTP levels include	Protein deficiency Hypothyroidism Malabsorption Kidney failure

Interfering Factors:

Falsely increased levels	Falsely decreased levels
• Men may present with high normal levels due to the large amounts of GGTP found in the prostate • Oral contraceptives	• Oral contraceptives

Related Tests:

SGPT/ALT, SGOT/AST, total serum bilirubin, serum ALP and ALP isoenzymes, serum LDH and LDH isoenzymes, total serum globulin, serum iron, serum ferritin, WBC and differential, EBV and CMV titers, hepatitis A, B, and C, mononucleosis, serum albumin, BUN, serum uric acid, serum and RBC magnesium

LDH

Background

Lactate dehydrogenase (LDH) is the enzyme that is involved in the catalytic conversion of pyruvate into lactate in the presence of NAD/NADH that occurs in every cell. Lactate is a major product of exercising muscle cells and red blood cell metabolism. Pyruvate is converted into lactate primarily under anaerobic conditions (some tissues and cell types also produce lactate under aerobic conditions). The lactate formed can be recycled. It is released into the blood stream and is eventually taken up by the liver. The liver converts it back into glucose, which is released back into the blood stream where it is taken up by muscles recovering from strenuous exercise, red blood cells, and other tissues.

Discussion

 LDH represents a group of enzymes that are involved in carbohydrate metabolism and the cellular transportation of chloride with glucose and glucose with zinc and sodium.

- Decreased levels of LDH often correspond to hypoglycemia (especially reactive hypoglycemia), pancreatic function, and glucose metabolism.

- Increased levels are used to evaluate the presence of tissue damage to the cell causing a rupture in the cellular cytoplasm.

- LDH is found in many of the tissues of the body, especially the heart, liver, kidney, skeletal muscle, brain, red blood cells, and lungs. Damage to any of these tissues will cause an elevated serum LDH level.

- The total LDH level is composed of fractions of 5 LDH isoenzymes. Each of these isoenzymes can be fractionated by electrophoresis into their constituent fraction.

- Since LDH is found in almost every tissue in the body, an elevated total LDH level has limited diagnostic value by itself. Anyone with a significantly increased total LDH level should have an LDH isoenzyme study performed to provide a more complete differential diagnosis.

Ranges:

	Standard U.S. Units	Standard International Units
Conventional Laboratory Range	1 – 240 U/L	1 – 240 U/L
Optimal Range	140 – 200 U/L	140 – 200 U/L
Alarm Ranges	<80 U/L or > 249 U/L	<80 U/L or > 249 U/L

When would you run this test?

1. To determine the presence of tissue damage

Clinical implications

HIGH

Clinical Implication	Additional information
Liver/Biliary dysfunction	If LDH is increased (>200) with increased total bilirubin (>1.2 or 20.5 µmol/dL), direct bilirubin (>0.2 or 3.4 µmol/dL), SGOT/AST (>30), GGTP (>30), and/or alkaline phosphatase (>100), liver/biliary dysfunction is **probable**.
	LDH is usually increased in liver congestion. Liver infection (hepatitis, infectious mononucleosis, EBV, CMV etc.) should be ruled out.
Cardiovascular disease	Elevated LDH levels are seen in cardiac dysfunction due to tissue stress and/or damage. Total LDH levels are elevated in about 90-95% of patients with acute MI. LDH levels become elevated about 24-48 hours after an MI.
	With a suspected MI, the SGOT/AST is increased 4-10 times above the reference range in acute myocardial infarct, peaking after 24 hours and normalizing after 3-4 days. Secondary rises in SGOT/AST levels suggest a recurring MI or continued infarction.
	Patients with a triglyceride level that is higher than the total cholesterol level and a decreased HDL (<55 or 1.42 mmol/L) have a higher risk for developing cardiovascular disease.
Anemia- B12/folate deficiency (megaloblastic)	Serum LDH levels are elevated in about 85% of those with megaloblastic anemia, which is primarily caused by a deficiency in vitamin B12 and/or folate. The megaloblastic changes cause an increased destruction of the red blood

	cells in the marrow, which is reflected in the increased LDH levels (>200). LDH can be used to help identify the **type** of anemia present. Isoenzyme fractionation typically shows an elevated LDH-1 In megaloblastic anemia. Other value changes seen with megaloblastic anemia include increased MCH (>31.2), MCV (>90), RDW (>13), serum iron (>100 or 17.91 µmol/dL) and decreased RBCs (<3.9 in women or 4.2 in men), and HGB (<13.5 or 135 g/L in women and <14 or 140 in men).
Anemia- hemolytic	Serum LDH levels are elevated (>200) in most people with hemolytic anemia. LDH levels can help assist in ruling out a hemolytic anemia. A normal LDH level with a substantial anemia seen in other values makes a hemolytic anemia less likely. An elevation of LDH-1 isoenzyme fraction that occurs with hemolytic anemia contributes to the increase in the total serum LDH value. In about 60% of hemolytic anemias the LDH-1 and LDH-2 fractions will be reversed, with a much higher LDH-2 level.
Non-specific tissue inflammation	An increased LDH level (>200) will be seen with non-specific tissue inflammation. Basophils will almost always be elevated (>3). During inflammation basophils deliver heparin to the effected tissue to prevent clotting. ESR will be increased along with a decreased serum albumin (<4.0 or 40g/L), total protein (<6.9 or 69 g/L), and globulin (<2.4 or 24 g/L).
Tissue destruction	As mentioned above any type of tissue destruction in the body will cause the rupture of the cell cytoplasm and the release of LDH. Damage and secondary inflammation will cause an increase in serum LDH. It is our recommendation that any patient who has an increase of more than 10 U/L above the reference range i.e. >240 U/L should have an LDH Isoenzyme fraction study to determine the exact location of the tissue damage. **Please see the section on LDH Isoenzymes on page 148 for further detail and interpretation.**
Viral infection 	LDH levels are usually elevated in about 95% of cases of infectious mononucleosis and Epstein Barr infection (EBV). LDH is usually elevated in cytomegalovirus infection (CMV). Other values usually take time to increase. **Pattern:** You may expect the following changes: decreased WBCs in first week, increased WBCs by 2nd week of illness, increased alkaline phosphatase and SGOT/AST (about 5-14 days after

	onset of illness), increased GGTP (about 7-21 days after onset of illness).	
Other conditions associated with increased LDH levels include	🐚 Hypothyroidism ⚕ Renal artery occlusion or embolism ⚕ Pulmonary infarction ⚕ Liver diseases ⚕ CHF	⚕ Malignant neoplasm ⚕ Skeletal muscle diseases ⚕ Sickle cell disease ⚕ Acute and chronic pancreatitis

LOW

Clinical Implication	Additional information
Reactive hypoglycemia	A common finding in reactive hypoglycemia is a decreased fasting blood glucose along with a decreased LDH (<140). Hemoglobin A1C levels may also be reduced (<4.1% or 0.057). LDH is an important enzyme for pyruvate metabolism in glycolysis and is associated with pancreatic function and glucose metabolism. Suspect hypoglycemia if there are also strong subjective indicators: 1. Strong craving for sweets (especially true for reactive hypoglycemia) 2. Awaken a few hours after sleeping, hard to get back to sleep 3. Crave coffee or sweets in the afternoon 4. Sleepy in the afternoon 5. Fatigue relieved by eating 6. Headache if meals are skipped or delayed 7. Irritable before meals 8. Shaky if meals are delayed Low blood pressure is a common finding with hypoglycemia and may be caused by adrenal insufficiency. A 5-6 hour oral glucose tolerance test with or without insulin levels may be necessary to determine if the patient is suffering from reactive hypoglycemia. If a glucose tolerance test is completed and there is evidence of a "flat curve", a heavy metal body burden is possible. Often with a heavy metal body burden or exposure to noxious gases, LDH-5 isoenzyme fraction will be decreased below 6%.

Interfering Factors:

Falsely increased levels	Falsely decreased levels
• Due to the high concentrations of LDH in red blood cells, abnormally elevated levels may occur if hemolysis occurs at time of the blood draw. • Strenuous exercise and muscular exertion • Skin diseases • Moderately increased in children <18 years of age • Pregnancy	• Some drugs

Related Tests:

LDH isoenzymes, Serum Alkaline phosphatase, alkaline phosphatase isoenzymes, serum CPK, SGPT/ALT, SGOT/AST, GGTP, Serum glucose, WBC and differential, RBC, RBC indices, total serum globulin, total protein, serum albumin, serum bilirubin, serum protein electrophoresis

LDH Isoenzymes

Discussion

The total LDH level is composed of fractions of 5 LDH isoenzymes. Each of these isoenzymes can be fractionated by electrophoresis into their constituent fraction. Anyone with a significantly increased total LDH level should have an LDH isoenzyme study performed. An increase in one or more of the isoenzymes is indicative of a destructive process in the specific tissue that correlates with the elevated isoenzymes. Early diagnosis can be made with an LDH isoenzyme study.

The tissue designations for LDH Isoenzymes

ISOENZYME	TISSUE
LDH-1	Heart, red blood cells
LDH-2	Heart, lymph, red blood cells
LDH-3	Pulmonary, spleen, adrenal, kidney, pancreas
LDH-4	Hepatic, skeletal muscle, prostate/uterus, skin
LDH-5	Hepatic, skeletal muscle, skin

Ranges: Expressed as a percentage of total serum LDH

		Reference Value:	Optimal value:
Conventional U.S. Range	LDH-1	22-36%	10-34%
	LDH-2	35-46%	30-45%
	LDH-3	13-26%	13-27%
	LDH-4	3-10%	2-14%
	LDH-5	2-12%	6-15%

When would you run this test?

1. This test is used in the differential diagnosis of acute MI, megaloblastic anemia due to vitamin B12, and/or folate deficiency, hemolytic anemia.

Clinical implications

HIGH

Clinical Implication	Additional information
Viral hepatitis	↑↑ LDH-4
Infectious mononucleosis	↑ LDH-1, LDH-2, LDH-3, LDH-5
Leukemia	↑ LDH-1, LDH-2, LDH-3, ↓ LDH-5
Vitamin B12/folic acid anemia	↑↑ LDH-1 and LDH-2 (rule out acute MI)
Acute MI	↑ LDH-1 equal or greater than LDH-2, ↑ LDH-5 (>18% increases the possibility)
Chronic and acute liver necrosis	↑ LDH-4, significantly ↑ LDH-5
Asthma	↑ LDH-3, ↑ LDH-5
Pulmonary embolism and infarction	Without bleeding into lungs: ↑ LDH-3 With bleeding into lungs: ↑ LDH-1, LDH-2, LDH-3
BPH/uterine hypertrophy	↑ LDH-4
Biliary obstruction-extra hepatic	↑ LDH-4, moderately ↑ LDH-5
Pancreatitis	↑ LDH-4
Adrenal cortical dysfunction	↑ LDH-3
Gall bladder disease	↑ LDH-3, LDH-5
Common bile duct dysfunction	↑ LDH-1, LDH-5

LOW

Clinical Implication	Additional information
Heavy metal body burden	↓ LDH-5 (< 6%)
Thyroid hypofunction secondary to anterior pituitary dysfunction (TSH <2.0)	↓ LDH –1 (<20%)
Exposure to noxious gases (Carbon monoxide etc.)	↓ LDH-5 (< 6%)

Interfering Factors:

Falsely increased levels	Falsely decreased levels
• None noted	• None noted

Related Tests:

Total LDH, Serum Alkaline phosphatase, alkaline phosphatase isoenzymes, serum CPK, SGPT/ALT, SGOT/AST, GGTP, Serum glucose, WBC and differential, RBC, RBC indices, total serum globulin, total protein, serum albumin, serum bilirubin, serum protein electrophoresis

Total Bilirubin

Background

Bilirubin is formed from the breakdown of hemoglobin from red blood cells, by the reticuloendothelial cells of the spleen and bone marrow. It is transported from these cells to the liver where it is conjugated (made water soluble) and excreted via the gall bladder in the bile. Increased serum levels of bilirubin occur with excessive red blood cell destruction or if there is a problem in the liver that prevents the normal excretion of bilirubin.

The total bilirubin is composed of two forms of bilirubin:

1. **Indirect or unconjugated bilirubin** is the protein (albumin) bound bilirubin that circulates in the blood on its way to the liver and ultimate conjugation. Elevated levels of indirect or unconjugated bilirubin are usually associated with increased red blood cell destruction.

2. **Direct or conjugated bilirubin** is the indirect or unconjugated bilirubin that has been conjugated with a number of different molecules, and then excreted in the bile. An increase in direct or conjugated bilirubin is usually associated with a dysfunction or blockage in the liver, gallbladder, or biliary tree.

Discussion

Total bilirubin is usually the only value reported on a standard chemistry screen. If the levels are elevated, consider ordering a differentiation of the total bilirubin, which will give you the conjugated and unconjugated values. We recommend obtaining the direct and indirect values on your routine chemistry screens. This will assist in determining if the cause of an increased total bilirubin is due to pre-hepatic situations (increased hemolysis) or post-hepatic problems (biliary obstruction etc.) If either the indirect or the direct has been reported, subtract that number from the total bilirubin and you will have the missing value.

An increased bilirubin level beyond the capacity of the liver to excrete it will lead to a visible staining of the tissue, called jaundice. The three major causes of jaundice are:

1. Hemolysis

2. Biliary obstruction outside the liver

3. Intra-hepatic biliary obstruction, which is usually due to injury to the cells of the liver (hepatitis, cirrhosis, infectious mononucleosis, drug reactions, etc.).

Ranges:

	Standard U.S. Units	Standard International Units
Conventional Laboratory Range	0.1 – 1.2 mg/dL	1.7 – 20.5 µmol/L
Optimal Range	0.1 – 1.2 mg/dL	1.7 – 20.5 µmol/L
Alarm Ranges	> 2.6 mg/dL	> 44.5 µmol/L

When would you run this test?

1. As part of a liver function panel
2. To investigate suspected biliary and liver dysfunction
3. To investigate suspected hemolysis

Clinical implications

HIGH

Clinical Implication	Additional information
Biliary stasis or insufficiency	Biliary stasis or insufficiency can often be caused by a mild obstruction in the extra-hepatic biliary duct. Bilirubin levels will be elevated (>1.2 or >20.5 µmol/dL) along with alkaline phosphatase (>100). GGTP, SGOT/AST, and SGPT/ALT may be normal or increased (>30). Many cases of biliary stasis will show normal lab values. In these situations suspect biliary stasis or insufficiency if there are strong subjective indicators: 1. Pain between shoulder blades 2. Stomach upset by greasy foods 3. Greasy or shiny stools 4. Nausea 5. Light or clay colored stools 6. Gallbladder attacks 7. Headache over the eye 8. Bitter taste in mouth, especially after meals
Oxidative stress	Oxidative stress can cause an increased destruction in red blood cells, which will cause an increased level of bilirubin. Free radical or oxidative stress is thought to be a major factor in many chronic illnesses. High levels of free radicals are associated with exposure to environmental pollutants, inflammatory diseases, and low antioxidant status. Free radicals are very unstable and reactive with other molecules.

	Once free radical reactions begin, they tend to multiply by chain reactions with cellular material. The chain reactions tend to have long lasting effects and the potential to cause cellular damage (i.e. cell membrane or DNA disruption). It is important to remember that our body needs a certain amount of oxidative stress to deal with toxins, microbes, etc. Both too much and too little oxidative stress is a problem. The Oxidata Free Radical test is an excellent in-office method of assessing oxidative stress.

Oxidata Free Radical Test

The Oxidata Free Radical Test determines the presence of free radical or oxidative stress and, by association, antioxidant status. The test measures the distal end of the polyunsaturated fat chain where aldehyde forms from free radical reaction. Aldehydes, present in many body compartments (serum, blood, etc.) are found in highest levels in urine. Urine aldehyde measurement is reportedly 50 times more sensitive than blood aldehyde levels. The test can help determine whether the oxidative activity is too low for optimal physiological function or whether the levels of oxidative stress are high, indicating free radical activity in the body.

Thymus dysfunction 	Consider an abnormality in the thymus with an elevated bilirubin (>1.2 or >20.5 μmol/dL) and increased HGB (>14.5 or 145 g/L in women or 15 or 150 g/L in men) , HCT (>44 or 0.44 in women and >48 or 0.48 in men), and RBCs (>4.5 in women and >4.9 in men) . Indications of thymus dysfunction include: 　1.　Delayed healing time 　2.　Immune insufficiency 　3.　Frequent colds and flu 　4.　Chemical sensitivity
Biliary tract obstruction (due to liver dysfunction) 	Conditions that cause damage to the liver cells (alcohol-induced injury, viral hepatitis, EBV, infectious mononucleosis, liver congestion, CMV) can cause obstruction in the small biliary channels between the liver cell groups that form the functional units of the liver and create a situation of liver dysfunction. Serum bilirubin levels will be elevated along with both conjugated and unconjugated fractions. The

	unconjugated fraction may be increased due to the liver's decreased ability to conjugate bilirubin due to liver cell damage. **Pattern:** Suspect biliary obstruction due to liver dysfunction when the total bilirubin is elevated (>1.2 or 20.5 μmol/dL) with increased GGTP (>30), SGPT/ALT (>30), alkaline phosphatase (>100), and/or LDH (>200). **Liver infection:** hepatitis, CMV, EBV, Infectious mono. etc. should be ruled out.
Biliary obstruction/ calculi	Bile duct obstruction/biliary calculi should be ruled out when total bilirubin is elevated (>1.2 or 20.5 μmol/dL) with an increased GGTP and a normal to increased SGPT/ALT. Direct and/or conjugated bilirubin levels will be elevated. A stone usually causes common bile duct obstruction. The level of total bilirubin increase is proportional to the degree of obstruction and how long the obstruction has been in place. **Pattern:** The total (>1.2 or 20.5 μmol/dL) and direct bilirubin (>0.2 or >5.4 μmol/dL) and GGTP (>30) will be increased and serum alkaline phosphatase will be significantly elevated (>140). The GGTP increase will be greater than the SGPT/ALT increase.
Liver dysfunction	An increased total bilirubin (>1.2 or 20.5 μmol/dL) is associated with liver dysfunction. Dysfunction in the liver may also cause an increase in SGPT/ALT (>30) from hepatocytes. Functionally oriented liver problems, such as detoxification issues, liver congestion, and conjugation problems are extremely common and should be evaluated based upon early prognostic indicators. The liver should always be viewed in the context of the hepato-biliary tree. Some of the key clinical indicators include: 1. Pain between shoulder blades 2. Stomach upset by greasy foods 3. If drinking alcohol, easily intoxicated 4. Headache over the eye 5. Sensitive to chemicals (perfume, cleaning solvents, insecticides, exhaust, etc.) 6. Hemorrhoids or varicose veins 7. Aggravated by coffee
RBC hemolysis	Increased hemolysis of red blood cells will lead to an

	increased formation of indirect or unconjugated bilirubin (>1.0 or 17.1 µmol/dL). The level of total bilirubin will rise when the level of indirect or unconjugated bilirubin exceeds the livers ability to clear it from the blood. The direct or conjugated fraction remains normal or slightly elevated.
	Hemolysis may be due to hemolytic anemia, autoimmune disease, Rh incompatibility, ABO incompatibility, and oxidative stress. RBC, HCT, HGB, MCV, MCH, MCHC, serum iron, TIBC, % transferrin saturation, and serum ferritin levels should be checked to differentiate anemia due to hemolysis.
Gilbert's syndrome	Gilbert's syndrome is a genetic defect in the ability to clear unconjugated or indirect bilirubin due to a decreased function in one of the phase II liver detoxification pathway enzymes. Males are affected more than females. Clinically, the disorder has elevated total bilirubin levels with 90% or more of the total bilirubin coming from unconjugated bilirubin. GGTP, SGOT/AST, and SGPT/ALT show no signs of abnormality. Diagnosis is difficult. Follow the patient for 12-18 months. Persistent elevated total and unconjugated bilirubin levels in the absence of other abnormal liver function tests is diagnostic for Gilbert's syndrome.
Other conditions associated with increased total bilirubin levels include	❋ Congestive heart failure ❋ Spleen dysfunction 🜚 Heavy metal body burden

LOW

Spleen insufficiency	A total bilirubin <0.1 or 1.7 µmol/dL, HGB <12.5 or 125 g/L and RBC <4.0, with serum iron > 100 or 17.91 µmol/dL suggests spleen insufficiency

Interfering Factors:

Falsely increased levels	Falsely decreased levels
• Prolonged fasting	• Exposure of sample to sunlight or bright artificial light at room temperature • High fat meal

Related Tests: GGTP, SGPT/ALT, SGOT/AST, Serum alkaline phosphatase, urinary bilirubin, urinary urobilinogen, RBC and indices, serum LDH

Direct (Conjugated) Bilirubin

Discussion

Direct or conjugated bilirubin is the indirect or unconjugated bilirubin that has been conjugated with a number of different molecules, and is then excreted in the bile. An increase in direct or conjugated bilirubin is usually associated with a dysfunction or blockage in the liver, gallbladder, or biliary tree.

Ranges:

	Standard U.S. Units	Standard International Units
Conventional Laboratory Range	0 – 0.2 mg/dL	0 – 3.4 µmol/L
Optimal Range	0 – 0.2 mg/dL	0 – 3.4 µmol/L
Alarm Ranges	> 0.8 mg/dL	>13.7 µmol/L

When would you run this test?

1. When the levels of total bilirubin are elevated to provide a differential diagnosis
2. To investigate suspected biliary and liver dysfunction
3. To investigate suspected hemolysis

Clinical implications

HIGH

Clinical Implication	Additional information
Biliary tract obstruction (due to liver dysfunction)	Conditions that cause damage to the liver cells (alcohol induced injury, viral hepatitis, EBV, infectious mononucleosis, liver congestion, CMV) can cause obstruction in the small biliary channels between the liver cell groups that form the functional units of the liver and create a situation of liver dysfunction. Serum bilirubin levels will be elevated along with both conjugated and unconjugated fractions. The unconjugated fraction may be increased due to the liver's decreased ability to conjugate bilirubin due to liver cell damage.

	Pattern: Suspect liver dysfunction when the total (>1.2 or 20.5 μmol/dL), direct (>0.2 or 3.4 μmol/dL), and indirect bilirubin (>1.0 or 17.1 μmol/dL) are elevated with increased GGTP (>30), SGPT/ALT (>30), alkaline phosphatase (>100), and/or LDH (>200). **Liver infections**: hepatitis, CMV, EBV, Infectious mono., etc. should be ruled out.
Bile duct obstruction (usually extra hepatic)/biliary calculi	Extra hepatic biliary duct obstruction will increase the level of direct or conjugated bilirubin since an obstruction outside the liver blocks the excretion of already conjugated bilirubin in the bile. Bile duct obstruction/biliary calculi should be ruled out when total bilirubin is >1.2 or 20.5 μmol/dL with an increased GGTP and a normal to increased SGPT/ALT. Direct or conjugated bilirubin levels will be elevated. A stone usually causes common bile duct obstruction. The level of total bilirubin increase is proportional to the degree of obstruction and how long the obstruction has been in place. **Pattern:** The total (>1.2 or 20.5 μmol/dL) and direct bilirubin (>0.2 or 3.4 μmol/dL), and GGTP (>30) will be increased; serum alkaline phosphatase (>140) will be significantly elevated. The GGTP increase will be greater than the SGPT/ALT increase.

LOW

Low levels of direct bilirubin have no clinical significance

Interfering Factors:

Falsely increased levels	Falsely decreased levels
• Prolonged fasting	• Exposure of sample to sunlight or bright artificial light at room temperature • High fat meal • Air bubble and shaking of sample

Related Tests: GGTP, SGPT/ALT, SGOT/AST, Serum alkaline phosphatase, urinary bilirubin, urinary urobilinogen, RBC and indices, serum LDH

Indirect (Unconjugated) Bilirubin

Discussion

 Indirect or unconjugated bilirubin is the protein (albumin) bound bilirubin that circulates in the blood on its way to the liver and ultimate conjugation. Elevated levels of indirect or unconjugated bilirubin are usually associated with increased red blood cell destruction.

Ranges:

	Standard U.S. Units	Standard International Units
Conventional Laboratory Range	0.1 – 1.0 mg/dL	1.7 – 17.1 µmol/L
Optimal Range	0.1 – 1.0 mg/dL	1.7 – 17.1 µmol/L
Alarm Ranges	> 1.8 mg/dL	>31 µmol/L

When would you run this test?

1. When the levels of total bilirubin are elevated to provide a differential diagnosis

2. To investigate suspected hemolysis

Clinical implications

HIGH

Clinical Implication	Additional information
RBC hemolysis	Increased hemolysis of red blood cells will lead to an increased formation of indirect or unconjugated bilirubin (>1.0 or 17.1 µmol/dL). The level of total bilirubin will rise when the level of indirect or unconjugated bilirubin exceeds the liver's ability to clear it from the blood. The direct or conjugated fraction remains normal or slightly elevated.
	Hemolysis may be due to hemolytic anemia, autoimmune disease, Rh incompatibility, ABO incompatibility, and oxidative

	stress. RBC, HCT, HGB, MCV, MCH, MCHC, serum iron, TIBC, % transferrin saturation, and serum ferritin levels should be checked to differentiate anemia due to hemolysis.
Gilbert's syndrome	Gilbert's syndrome is a genetic defect in the ability to clear unconjugated or indirect bilirubin due to a decreased function in one of the phase II liver detoxification pathway enzymes. Males are affected more than females. Clinically, the disorder has elevated total bilirubin levels with 90% or more of the total bilirubin coming from unconjugated bilirubin. GGTP SGOT/AST, and SGPT/ALT show no signs of abnormality. Diagnosis is difficult. Follow the patient for 12-18 months. Persistently elevated total and unconjugated bilirubin level in the absence of other abnormal liver function tests is diagnostic for Gilbert's syndrome.
Other conditions associated with increased levels of indirect bilirubin include	✳ Trauma ✳ Large hematomas, ✳ Hemorrhagic pulmonary infarcts ✳ Excessive red blood cell production (pernicious anemia, severe lead poisoning)

LOW

Low levels of indirect bilirubin have no clinical significance

Interfering Factors:

Falsely increased levels	Falsely decreased levels
• Prolonged fasting	• Exposure of sample to sunlight or bright artificial light at room temperature • High fat meal • Air bubble and shaking of sample

Related Tests:

GGTP, SGPT/ALT, SGOT/AST, Serum alkaline phosphatase, urinary bilirubin, urinary urobilinogen, EB and indices, serum LDH

Total Serum Iron

Background

70% of the iron in the body is in the form of hemoglobin. The remaining 30% is found in storage form in the liver, spleen, and bone marrow. The average intake of iron is about 10 mg/day, and only about 10% is absorbed. Iron is best absorbed when taken about 45-50 minutes away from food. Dairy products, foods with high fiber contents, coffee, tea, and meat inhibit absorption. Vitamin C enhances absorption.

The majority of body iron comes from dietary sources in the form of ferric iron, which has to be reduced into ferrous iron after ingestion in order to be absorbed, a process that requires stomach acid and vitamin C. Iron is absorbed primarily in the duodenum and jejunum. Once absorbed, iron travels in the blood attached to a beta globulin molecule called transferrin. The RBC precursors in the bone marrow use a large proportion of the iron. About 60% of the remainder is stored in the bone marrow, liver, and spleen as ferritin, and 40% as hemosiderin.

Discussion

The serum iron measurement reflects iron bound to serum protein, the most predominant of which is transferrin and at any one time about 1/3rd of the transferrin is saturated with iron. Serum iron relies both on the quantity of iron present and the amount of transferrin available. Serum iron levels will begin to fall somewhere between the depletion of the iron stores and the development of anemia.

- Many physicians make the mistake of only ordering RBC and indices when investigating iron excess or iron deficiency anemia. Without the total serum iron and other iron tests, such as ferritin, TIBC, and % transferrin saturation, the degree of iron deficiency anemia or iron excess cannot be appreciated.

- Ordering serum iron without a serum ferritin and TIBC has very little clinical value.

- Diurnal variations in serum iron levels have been noted. The peak value occurs most often in the morning.

Ranges:

	Standard U.S. Units	Standard International Units
Conventional Laboratory Range	30 – 170 µg/dL	5.37 – 30.45 µmol/L
Optimal Range	50 – 100 µg/dL	8.96 – 17.91 µmol/L
Alarm Ranges	<25 or >200 µg/dL	<4.5 or > 35.82 µmol/L

When would you run this test?

1. To assess for iron deficiency anemia
2. To monitor iron deficiency anemia treatment
3. To monitor conditions of iron overload

Clinical implications

HIGH

Clinical Implication	Additional information
Liver dysfunction	A high serum iron (> 100 or 17.91 µmol/dL) may be a sign of liver dysfunction. If the serum iron is increased along with increased liver enzymes, liver dysfunction is **probable**. Functionally oriented liver problems, such as detoxification issues, liver congestion, and conjugation problems are extremely common and should be evaluated based upon early prognostic indicators. The liver should always be viewed in the context of the hepato-biliary tree. Some of the key clinical indicators include: 1. Pain between shoulder blades 2. Stomach upset by greasy foods 3. If drinking alcohol, easily intoxicated 4. Headache over the eye 5. Sensitive to chemicals (perfume, cleaning solvents, insecticides, exhaust, etc.) 6. Hemorrhoids or varicose veins
Hemochromatosis/ hemosiderosis/iron overload	Hemochromatosis is a disease produced by an excess absorption of iron, which leads to deposition of excess iron in the tissues, especially the liver. • **Hemochromatosis** refers to the hereditary iron

storage disorder

- **Hemosiderosis** refers to the non-hereditary form.

Hemochromatosis is more common in males, with a clinical onset between the ages of 40-60. The disease can lead to cirrhosis, diabetes, liver enlargement, and bronzing of skin.

Pattern:

Laboratory changes include an increased serum iron (>220 or 39.40 μmol/dL)), a decreased TIBC (<250 or 44.8 μmol/dL), an increased % transferrin saturation (usually > 60%), and an increased ferritin level (often >1000 μg/dL). SGOT/AST is usually elevated (>40).

All family members of the patient diagnosed with hereditary hemochromatosis should be screened for the problem. The problem is often silent (no symptoms); however, it will almost always result (if not corrected) in heart disease, liver/biliary disease, bacterial infection, dementia, atherosclerosis, diabetes, or stroke. If dietary and supplemental support is not successful, patient should be referred for phlebotomy and/or deferoxamine chelation.

Excess consumption of iron

Excess consumption of iron can come from a number of different sources:

- Elevated levels of iron in the drinking water

- Iron cookware, especially when used to cook acidic foods e.g. tomatoes

- Consumption of iron containing supplements

All of the above are often the reason for an increased serum iron or ferritin. These causes of an increased serum iron should be ruled out before hemochromatosis/iron overload is assumed.

Iron conversion problem	If the serum iron is normal or increased (>100 or 17.91 μmol/dL) with a decreased RBC (<3.9 in women or 4.2 in men) , HGB (<13.5 or 135 g/L in women and <14 or 140 g/L in men), or HCT (<37 or 0.37 in women and 40 or 0.4 in men), consider that there may be an inability of the body to convert inorganic iron (the type found in serum iron) into hemoglobin (organic iron). There is probably a need for B12, folic acid, B6, and/or copper

Viral infection	If serum iron is increased (100 or 17.91 μmol/dL) along with an increased (>7.5), or decreased (<5.0) WBC count and a decreased lymphocyte count (<24), the reason for this pattern may be a long term viral infection.	
Other conditions associated with increased total serum iron levels include	Spleen dysfunction (if bilirubin levels are elevated) Poor utilization of iron Iron conversion anemias (vitamin B12, folic acid, B6, copper, molybdenum deficiency)	Viral hepatitis Thalassemia Lead poisoning Renal dysfunction Hemolytic anemia Pernicious anemia

To receive master copies of our tracking forms and conversion tables please visit:

www.BloodChemistryAnalysis.com

If you're interested in a software program to help with your analysis please visit:
www.BloodChemSoftware.com

LOW

Clinical Implication	Additional information
Anemia- iron deficiency	This is the most prevalent anemia worldwide. The major causes are: 1. Dietary inadequacies & Malabsorption 2. Increased iron loss 3. Increased iron requirements e.g. pregnancy **Patterns:** If there is a decreased serum iron (< 50 or 8.96 μmol/dL) with a decreased MCH (<28), MCV (<82), and MCHC (<32), ferritin (<33 in men and 10 in women), % transferrin saturation and/or HGB (<13.5 or 135 g/L in women and <14 or 140 in men) and/or HCT (<37 or 0.37 in women and 40 or 0.4 in men), and increased RDW (>13), then iron deficiency anemia is **probable**.

	✻ If TIBC is increased (>350 or 62.7 μmol/dL), internal/microscopic bleeding is **possible**, and should be ruled out with reticulocyte count, urinalysis, and/or stool analysis.
	🌰 If serum phosphorous is decreased (<3.0 or <0.97 mmol/L) and serum globulin is increased (>2.8 or 28 g/L) or decreased (<2.4 or 24 g/L), iron anemia may be **secondary to hypochlorhydria**.
	Some of the subjective indicators for iron need are: 1. Prolonged fatigue, particularly in pregnancy 2. Blue sclera of the eyes 3. Pica and a desire to chew ice 4. Inability to tolerate cold
Hypochlorhydria 	A low serum iron level is often associated with hypochlorhydria. Adequate levels of stomach acid are necessary for iron absorption. **Pattern:** 🌰 Hypochlorhydria is **possible** with a low serum iron (< 50 or 8.96 μmol/dL) and an increased (> 2.8 or 28 g/L) or decreased (<2.4 or 24 g/L) total globulin. 🌰 Hypochlorhydria is **probable** if the BUN is also increased (>16 or 5.71 mmol/L) and/or serum phosphorous is decreased (<3.0 or <0.97 mmol/L). **Please see the special topic on hypochlorhydria on page 96 for more details.**
Internal bleeding and internal microscopic bleeding 	A decreased total serum iron (< 50 or 8.96 μmol/dL) may be due to internal bleeding. TIBC (>350 or 62.7 μmol/dL), transferrin, and reticulocyte count (>1) will be elevated. HGB (<13.5 or 135 g/L in women and <14 or 140 in men) and HCT (<37 or 0.37 in women and 40 or 0.4 in men) may be decreased or normal depending on the severity of the bleeding. Internal microscopic bleeding may present with a decreased TIBC (<250 or 44.8 μmol/dL) and an elevated reticulocyte count. If this pattern is present, internal bleeding **must** be ruled out with reticulocyte count, urinalysis, and/or stool analysis. **Refer to a doctor qualified to diagnose and treat internal bleeding.**

Other conditions associated with decreased total serum iron levels include	✤ Infection ✤ Increased blood loss during menses 🥚 Free radical pathology 🥚 Vitamin C need	✤ Renal dysfunction ✤ Chronic renal failure 🥚 Hypothyroidism 🥚 Liver dysfunction

Interfering Factors:

The treatment of megaloblastic or vitamin B12/folate deficiency anemia can cause a temporary fall in serum iron. This is due to the increased utilization of previously available but unused iron.

Falsely increased levels	Falsely decreased levels
• Drugs: estrogens, oral contraceptives • Alcohol consumption	• None noted

Related Tests:

RBC, HGB, HCT, MCV, MCH, serum ferritin, TIBC, % transferrin saturation, reticulocyte count, total serum globulin (HCL need)

Serum Ferritin

Discussion

 Ferritin is the main storage form of iron in the body. Decreased serum ferritin levels parallel tissue ferritin levels, which in turn reflects the decreased iron storage found in iron deficiency anemia. In most situations the serum ferritin level will occur before changes in serum iron, development of anemia, or changes in RBC morphology. The body will do whatever it takes to keep the serum levels of iron at an optimal level. Ferritin is the most sensitive test to detect iron deficiency.

Ranges:

Ferritin will usually be increased in adult men after 50 and women after menopause.

	Reference and optimal value:	Alarm ranges:
Conventional U.S. Range	**Males**: 33 – 236 ng/ml **Females**: Before menopause: 10 – 122 ng/ml After menopause: 10 – 263 ng/ml	< 8 ng/dL > 500 ng/dL
Standard International Units	**Males**: 33-236 µg/L **Females**: Before menopause: 10 – 122 µg/L After menopause: 10 – 263 µg/L	< 8 µg/L > 500 µg/L

When would you run this test?

1. To assess for iron deficiency anemia

2. To monitor iron deficiency anemia treatment

3. To monitor conditions of iron overload

Clinical implications

HIGH

Clinical Implication	Additional information
Hemochromatosis/ hemosiderosis/iron overload	Hemochromatosis is a disease produced by an excess absorption of iron, which leads to deposition of excess iron in the tissues, especially the liver. • **Hemochromatosis** refers to the hereditary iron storage disorder

	• **Hemosiderosis** refers to the non-hereditary form. Hemochromatosis is more common in males, with a clinical onset between the ages of 40-60. The disease can lead to cirrhosis, diabetes, liver enlargement, and bronzing of skin. **Pattern:** Laboratory changes include an increased serum iron (>220 or 39.40 µmol/dL), a decreased TIBC (<250 or 44.8 µmol/dL), an increased % transferrin saturation (usually > 60%), and **an increased ferritin level (often >1000 µg/dL)**. SGOT/AST is usually elevated (>40). All family members of the patient diagnosed with hereditary hemochromatosis should be screened for the problem. The problem is often silent (no symptoms); however, it will almost always result (if not corrected) in heart disease, liver/biliary disease, bacterial infection, dementia, atherosclerosis, diabetes, or stroke. If dietary and supplemental support is not successful, patient should be referred for phlebotomy and/or deferoxamine chelation.
Excess consumption of iron	Excess consumption of iron can come from a number of different sources: • Elevated levels of iron in the drinking water • Iron cookware, especially when used to cook acidic foods e.g. tomatoes • Consumption of iron containing supplements All of the above are often the reason for an increased serum iron or ferritin
Inflammation/ liver dysfunction/ oxidative stress	Serum ferritin is one of a group of proteins that can become increased in response to inflammation, infection, or trauma. Elevations can last for weeks. **Pattern:** An elevated ferritin (>236 in men and 122 in women) along with normal serum iron is suggestive of inflammation, liver dysfunction, or oxidative stress.
Other conditions associated with increased serum ferritin levels include	Blood transfusions Chronic hepatitis Megaloblastic/B12/folate deficiency anemia Chronic renal disease Hemolytic anemia

LOW

Clinical Implication	Additional information
Anemia- iron deficiency	**Patterns** ✳ If ferritin is decreased (<33 in men and 10 in women) along with decreased serum iron (< 50 or 8.96 µmol/dL) and % transferrin saturation, iron anemia is **probable**. This can be confirmed with a CBC, which will show a decreased RBC count (<3.9 in women or 4.2 in men), MCH (<28), MCV (<82), MCHC (<32), and/or HGB (<13.5 or 135 g/L in women and <14 or 140 in men) HCT (<37 or 0.37 in women and 40 or 0.4 in men) , and increased RDW (>13). ✳ If TIBC is increased (>350 or 62.7µmol/dL), microscopic bleeding is **possible**, and should be ruled out with reticulocyte count, urinalysis, and/or stool analysis. 🍋 If serum phosphorous is decreased (<3.0 or <0.97 mmol/L) and serum globulin is increased (>2.8 or 28 g/L) or decreased (<2.4 or 24 g/L), iron anemia may be secondary to hypochlorhydria. Some of the subjective indicators for iron need are: 1. Prolonged fatigue, particularly in pregnancy 2. Blue sclera of the eyes 3. Pica and a desire to chew ice 4. Inability to tolerate cold

Interfering Factors:

Falsely increased levels	Falsely decreased levels
• None noted	• None noted

Related Tests:

RBC, HGB, HCT, MCV, MCH, TIBC, Serum total iron, reticulocyte count, Oxidata free radical test, SGOT/AST, SGPT/ALT, GGTP

Total Iron Binding Capacity

Discussion

Total Iron Binding Capacity is an approximate estimation of the serum transferrin level. Transferrin is the protein that carries the majority of the iron in the blood. TIBC is not an exact measurement of transferrin because not all of the iron is bound by transferrin. The test is performed by saturating the serum with excess iron, which saturates the transferrin present in the sample. From this reading you can estimate the capacity for the transferrin to bind iron. All the iron not bound to protein is removed and the serum iron is measured.

Ranges:

	Standard U.S. Units	Standard International Units
Conventional Laboratory Range	250 – 350 µg/dL	44.8 – 62.7 µmol/L
Optimal Range	250 – 350 µg/dL	44.8 – 62.7 µmol/L

When would you run this test?

1. To assess for iron deficiency anemia
2. To monitor iron deficiency anemia treatment
3. To monitor conditions of iron overload

Clinical implications

HIGH

Clinical Implication	Additional information
Anemia- iron deficiency	If the total iron binding capacity is increased (>350 or 62.7 µmol/dL) along with a decreased total iron (< 50 or 8.96 µmol/dL), MCV (<82), MCH (<28), Serum ferritin (< 33 in men and 10 in women), % transferrin saturation, and/or HGB (<13.5 or 135 g/L in women and <14 or 140 in men) and/or HCT (<37 or 0.37 in women and 40 or 0.4 in men) , iron anemia is **probable**.

Internal bleeding	With a high (>350 or 62.7 μmol/dL) TIBC there is always the possibility of microscopic bleeding, which should be ruled out with reticulocyte count, urinalysis, and/or stool analysis.	
Other conditions associated with increased TIBC levels include	❀ Late pregnancy ❀ Liver dysfunction	❀ Hepatitis ❀ Blood loss

LOW

Clinical Implication	Additional information
Hemochromatosis/ hemosiderosis/iron overload	Hemochromatosis is a disease produced by an excess absorption of iron, which leads to deposition of excess iron in the tissues, especially the liver. • **Hemochromatosis** refers to the hereditary iron storage disorder • **Hemosiderosis** refers to the non-hereditary form. Hemochromatosis is more common in males, with a clinical onset between the ages of 40-60. The disease can lead to cirrhosis, diabetes, liver enlargement, and bronzing of the skin. **Pattern** Laboratory changes include an increased serum iron (>220 or 39.40μmol/dL), a decreased TIBC (<250 or 44.8 μmol/dL), an increased % transferrin saturation (usually > 60%), and an increased ferritin level (often >1000 μg/dL). SGOT/AST is usually elevated (>40). All family members of the patient diagnosed with hereditary hemochromatosis should be screened for the problem. The problem is often silent (no symptoms); however, it will almost always result (if not corrected) in heart disease, liver/biliary disease, bacterial infection, dementia, atherosclerosis, diabetes, or stroke. If dietary and supplemental support is not successful, patient should be referred for phlebotomy and/or deferoxamine chelation.
Microscopic bleeding	The probability of microscopic internal bleeding is high if the TIBC is decreased along with an increased reticulocyte count. **This patient should be referred to a doctor qualified to diagnose and treat internal bleeding.**

Diet- protein malnutrition	Conditions of low protein in the body, such as malnutrition, starvation, nephrotic syndrome, or cancer, can cause a decreased level of TIBC (<250 or 44.8 μmol/dL).	
Other conditions associated with decreased TIBC levels include	❋ Chronic inflammatory disorders 🫀 Liver dysfunction	❋ Thalassemia ❋ Hyperthyroidism

Interfering Factors:

Falsely increased levels	Falsely decreased levels
• Oral contraceptives	• None noted

Related Tests:

RBC, HGB, HCT, MCV, MCH, serum ferritin, serum total iron, reticulocyte count

% Transferrin Saturation

Background

The % saturation index is a calculated value that is a better index of iron saturation than transferrin levels by themselves. It is also said to be a more sensitive screening test for iron deficiency than either serum iron or TIBC alone.

Discussion

The classic pattern of iron deficiency shows a decreased serum iron and an increased TIBC. This will increase the unsaturated binding capacity of transferrin and decrease the percent of transferrin bound to iron. A % transferrin saturation of 15% or below is a classic finding in iron deficiency anemia. The % transferrin saturation is calculated using the following formula:

% transferrin saturation = (Serum iron X 100) / TIBC

Ranges:

	Reference Value:	Optimal value:	Alarm ranges:
Conventional U.S. Range	16 – 60%	20 – 35%	< 5% > 70%

When would you run this test?

1. Differential diagnosis of anemia

2. Assessment and following the treatment for iron deficiency anemia

Clinical implications

HIGH

Clinical Implication	Additional information
Hemochromatosis/ hemosiderosis/iron overload	Hemochromatosis is a disease produced by an excess absorption of iron, which leads to deposition of excess iron in the tissues, especially the liver.

	• **Hemochromatosis** refers to the hereditary iron storage disorder • **Hemosiderosis** refers to the non-hereditary form. Hemochromatosis is more common in males, with a clinical onset between the ages of 40-60. The disease can lead to cirrhosis, diabetes, liver enlargement, and bronzing of the skin. **Pattern:** Laboratory changes include an increased serum iron (>220 or 39.40 µmol/dL), a decreased TIBC (<250 or 44.8 µmol/dL), an increased % transferrin saturation (usually > 60%), and an increased ferritin level (often >1000 µg/dL). SGOT/AST is usually elevated (>40). All family members of the patient diagnosed with hereditary hemochromatosis should be screened for the problem. The problem is often silent (no symptoms); however, it will almost always result (if not corrected) in heart disease, liver/biliary disease, bacterial infection, dementia, atherosclerosis, diabetes, or stroke. If dietary and supplemental support is not successful, patient should be referred for phlebotomy and/or deferoxamine chelation.

Other conditions associated with increased % transferrin saturation levels include	✳ Hemolytic anemia ✳ Megaloblastic anemia ✳ Iron overload ✳ Thalassemia 🌰 Protein malnutrition	✳ Cirrhosis ✳ Lead poisoning 🌰 B12 and/or folate deficiency 🌰 B6 deficiency

LOW

Clinical Implication	Additional information	
Anemia- iron deficiency	If the total iron binding capacity is increased (>350 or 62.7 µmol/dL) along with a decreased total iron (< 50 or 8.96 µmol/dL), MCV (<82), MCH (<28), Serum ferritin (<33 in men and 10 in women), % transferrin saturation and/or HGB (<13.5 or 135 g/L in women and 14 or 140 in men) and/or HCT (<37 or 0.37 in women and 40 or 0.4 in men) , iron anemia is **probable**.	
Other conditions associated with decreased %	✳ Anemia of chronic disease ✳ Chronic infection	✳ Pregnancy in 3rd trimester 🌰 B12 or folate deficiency

transferrin saturation levels include	✳ Uremia, malignancies	with concomitant iron deficiency
	✳ Tissue inflammation	

Related Tests:

RBC, HGB, HCT, MCV, MCH, serum ferritin, serum iron, TIBC, reticulocyte count, total serum globulin (HCL need)

Serum Iron, TIBC and % Transferrin Saturation patterns

The patterns seen between serum iron, TIBC and % Transferrin Saturation levels can be quite useful diagnostically.

Serum Iron	TIBC	% TS	Clinical Implication
↓	↓	↓	• Chronic infection • Uremia • Malignancies • Rheumatoid-collagen disorders and tissue inflammation
↓	↑	↓	• Chronic iron deficiency anemia • Pregnancy in 3rd trimester
↓	↓	Normal or ↑	• Protein malnutrition • Nephrotic syndrome • Cirrhosis
↑	↓	↑	• Hemochromatosis • Iron overload (usually from therapy) • Hemolytic anemia • Lead poisoning • B12 and/or folate deficiency • B6 deficiency
↑	↑	Normal	• Oral contraceptives • Acute hepatitis
↑	Normal or ↓	Normal or ↑	• B12 and/or folate deficiency
↓	Normal	↓	• Acute infection • Chronic iron deficiency
Normal	↑	↓	• B12 and/or folate deficiency with concomitant iron deficiency

TSH

Background

Thyroid hormone synthesis and secretion is regulated via a negative feed-back control system, which involves the hypothalamus, anterior pituitary, and the thyroid gland. Thyrotrophin-releasing hormone (TRH) is secreted by the hypothalamus. TRH stimulates the anterior pituitary to secrete TSH, which acts on the thyroid gland to stimulate the release of T-3 and T-4. T-3 and T-4 act negatively on the anterior pituitary gland to suppress the release of TSH, thereby controlling thyroid hormone production.

Discussion

 TSH is the most sensitive test for primary hypothyroidism. However if there is a clinical picture of hypothyroidism, yet the TSH is normal then investigate other causes within the thyroid-pituitary-hypothalamic feedback axis.

● With normal thyroid and anterior pituitary/hypothalamus function, a decreased T-3 and T-4 causes an increase in TSH, and an increase in T-3 and T-4 causes a decrease in TSH.

● TSH is an integral part of a thyroid panel useful for the determination and potential differentiation of hypothyroidism.

● TSH is used to diagnose primary hypothyroidism when there is a problem intrinsic to the thyroid gland itself. TSH levels will be elevated.

● When TSH levels are decreased the problem may be reflective of a hyperthyroid state. Also consider that the problem may be due to abnormalities outside the thyroid in the pituitary-hypothalamic axis, which cause a secondary and even tertiary hypothyroidism.

● Although sensitive it is not uncommon for a patient with a clinical picture of hypothyroidism to have completely normal serum thyroid tests. In these cases this should alert the clinician to an etiology other than an intrinsic thyroid gland dysfunction (i.e. increased tissue resistance to thyroid hormone.) Consider other low T-3 or low T-4 syndromes, such as subclinical hypothyroidism and Wilson's syndrome. **Please see the special topic on Wilson's syndrome on page 188 for more information**.

Ranges:

	Standard U.S. Units	Standard International Units
Conventional Laboratory Range	0.35 – 5.5 µIU/ml	0.35 – 5.5 mIU/l
Optimal Range	2.0 – 4.4 µIU/ml	2.0 – 4.4 mIU/l
Alarm Ranges	< 0.3 or > 10.0 µIU/ml	< 0.3 or > 10.0 mIU/l

When would you run this test?

1. To identify the cause of a thyroid related problem
2. As part of a thyroid screening panel

Clinical implications

HIGH

Clinical Implication	Additional information
Primary hypothyroidism	Hypothyroidism is a very common and often undiagnosed condition. Individual blood indices are notoriously insensitive to mild or borderline cases of primary hypothyroidism. In many cases TSH levels may be within normal limits yet the patient is suffering from all the classic signs and symptoms of low thyroid. In these cases it is often more efficacious to look at more functional criteria such as basal body temperature, Achilles return reflex, and iodine status, along with history, other blood indices, and clinical signs and symptoms. **Please see the special topic on functional tests for hypothyroidism below.** Pattern: If TSH levels are elevated (> 4.4), with a normal or decreased T-4 level (<6 or 7.2 nmol/L) and/or T-3 (<100 or 1.54 nmol/L), a decreased T-3 uptake (<27), and an increased cholesterol (>220 or 5.69 mmol/L) and triglyceride level (>110 or 1.24 mmol/L), primary hypothyroidism is **probable**. Some of the clinical signs of hypothyroidism include:

	1. Difficulty losing weight
	2. Mentally sluggish, reduced initiative
	3. Easily fatigued, sleepy during the day
	4. Sensitive to cold, poor circulation (cold hands and feet)
	5. Constipation, chronic
	6. Excessive hair loss and / or coarse hair
	7. Morning headaches, wear off during the day
	8. Loss of lateral 1/3 of eyebrow
	9. Seasonal sadness

 # Functional Tests for Hypothyroidism

1. Achilles return reflex

- A delayed Achilles return reflex is a classic sign of hypothyroidism.

- In the absence of spinal lesions, a delayed Achilles return reflex bilaterally indicates the strong likelihood for low thyroid activity, along with the corresponding signs and symptoms.

2. Basal Body Temperature test

- The basal body temperature (BBT) reflects the body's basal metabolism, which refers to the amount of energy your body burns at rest.

- The basal metabolism is largely determined by hormones secreted from the thyroid and to a lesser degree the adrenal glands.

- The function of the thyroid can be observed by measuring the fluctuations of the basal body temperature over a number of days.

- Reduced axillary temperature is also common with reduced adrenal function, a diet low in essential fatty acids, protein malnutrition and thiamine deficiency. Therefore, you should not equivocally associate a depressed temperature with a pure thyroid problem.

3. Iodine skin test

- The iodine skin test is a functional assessment for iodine status in the body.

- By painting the skin with a 2% solution of iodine we can see how quickly the body absorbs the available iodine.

- The quicker the iodine fades, the greater the deficiency can be assumed to be.

Drug causes of ↑	✳ Prescription Lithium therapy	
	✳ Potassium iodide	
	✳ TSH injections	
Other conditions associated with increased TSH levels include	✳ Hashimoto's thyroiditis	✳ Severe debilitating illness
	✳ Sub acute thyroiditis	✳ Thyrotoxicosis
	🖐 Liver/biliary dysfunction due to conjugation problems	✳ Thyrotropin producing tumor

LOW

Clinical Implication	Additional information
Hyperthyroidism	Although less common than hypothyroidism, the following pattern may help elucidate a developing or existent hyperthyroid state.
	Pattern:
	If TSH is low (<2.0) with an increased T-3 (>230 or 3.53 nmol/L), T-3 uptake (>37), FTI and/or T-4 (>12 or 154.4 nmol/L), then hyperthyroidism is **probable**. Consider running thyroid antibody studies to rule out Hashimoto's thyroiditis and Grave's disease. **Please see the special topic below for more details on thyroid antibody studies.**
	Rule-out food allergy/sensitivities, environmental sensitivities, recent immunizations/inoculations, viral infections, and other auto-immune problems in any cases of suspected hyperthyroidism. Some of the clinical signs of hyperthyroidism include:
	1. Difficulty gaining weight, even with large appetite
	2. Nervous, emotional, can't work under pressure
	3. Inward trembling
	4. Flush easily
	5. Fast pulse at rest
	6. Intolerance to high temperatures

Thyroid Antibody Studies

Consider running anti-thyroid antibody studies (i.e. anti-thyroglobulin antibody, thyroid anti-microsomal and thyroid peroxidase antibody) with known or suspected thyroid abnormality. Differentiation between multiple auto-immune conditions (i.e. Hashimoto's, Grave's disease and sub-acute thyroiditis) is based upon these antibody titers. With Hashimoto's and Grave's disease the titers will be significantly elevated. With sub-acute thyroiditis, the levels are usually slightly increased.

Secondary Hypothyroidism **(Anterior Pituitary Hypofunction)**	Thyroid hypofunction is often secondary to an anterior pituitary hypofunction (*Secondary Hypothyroidism*). If the subjective indications of thyroid hypofunction are present along with a decreased T-3 uptake (<27) and normal T-4, T-3, and FTI, with the TSH <2.0, **Anterior Pituitary Hypofunction** should be considered. If serum triglycerides are elevated (>110 or 1.24 mmol/L) and the total cholesterol levels are decreased (<150 or 3.9 mmol/L), then secondary hypothyroidism is **probable**. Anterior pituitary hypofunction is a common problem and one that is frequently mistaken for thyroid hypofunction (the subjective indications are usually identical and the patient's axillary temperature will frequently be below normal). Some of the common clinical indications of an anterior pituitary dysfunction include: 1. Decreased libido 2. Weight gain around hips or waist 3. Menstrual irregularities 4. Delayed sexual development (after age 13) 5. Unresponsive thyroid treatment 6. Hypoglycemia due to concomitant adrenal insufficiency
Tertiary hypothyroidism **(Hypothalamus hypofunction)**	A decreased TSH level (<2.0) may be due to an inadequate secretion of Thyroid Releasing Hormone (TRH) from the hypothalamus. Please see the special topic below on the differentiation of hypothyroid classification for more details.
Heavy metal body burden (e.g. lead,	Consider a heavy metal body burden with a thyroid condition that is unresponsive to treatment. Specific metals include

aluminum, cadmium and other toxic metals)	aluminum, mercury, and cadmium that act as disruptors to thyroid receptor activity. Other standard laboratory signs useful in elucidating a potential heavy metal body burden include MCHC, MCH, and uric acid.	
	One of the significant effects of toxic metals is the impact they have on red blood cells especially hemoglobin. If MCH (<28) and MCHC (<32) is decreased with a decreased uric acid (<3.5 or 208 μmol/dL), suspect a heavy metal body burden. Confirm with a hair analysis or toxic element testing via blood or urine. The serum levels of the metals may also be increased, but in sub-acute conditions the serum levels may be normal. The hair and urinary/blood tests will frequently reflect the increase before it is seen outside the reference range in the serum.	
Drug causes of ⬇	✣ T-3 treatment ✣ Aspirin ✣ Corticosteroids	✣ Heparin ✣ Dopamine
Other conditions associated with decreased TSH levels include	🫘 Protein malnutrition ✣ Hashimoto's thyroiditis	✣ Pregnancy ✣ Sub acute thyroiditis

Differentiation of hypothyroid classifications

A decreased TSH level may be due to an inadequate secretion of Thyroid Releasing Hormone (TRH) from the hypothalamus. Clinically an intravenous injection of TRH is administered to try to stimulate the production of TSH from the pituitary.

✣ In **primary hypothyroidism** there is an exaggerated TSH response after administration of TRH.

✣ In **secondary hypothyroidism** due to anterior pituitary hypofunction there is no significant rise in TSH levels after administration of TRH.

✣ In **tertiary hypothyroidism** due to a hypothalamic hypofunction there will be a delayed rise in TSH of approximately 30 minutes after administration of TRH.

Interfering Factors:

Falsely increased levels	Falsely decreased levels
• Administration of radioisotopes within one week prior to testing • Please see drug causes of increase above	• Please see drug causes of decrease above

Related Tests:

T-3 uptake, thyroxine (T-4), free thyroxine index , thyroid binding globulin (TBG), serum triglycerides, serum cholesterol, thyrotrophin releasing hormone (TRH), serum calcium, serum phosphorous, serum potassium, serum sodium, RBC magnesium, HCT, HGB, serum albumin

Considerations when Interpreting a Thyroid Test or Panel

- The thyroid is a complex endocrine gland that works in concert with many other endocrine glands with hormonal mediators. Support the whole system as well as the specific organ or gland.

- When addressing any endocrine dysfunction, **always support the key essentials** to normal function first (nutritional deficiencies, fatty acid metabolism, protein/albumin availability, liver activity, hidden infections etc.).

- **Liver conjugation** problems can significantly impair hormone levels from the thyroid, gonads, or adrenal cortex. Therefore, attention should be paid to optimizing liver function prior to exhausting specific endocrine causes or treatments.

- Thyroid hormone activity, along with other hormones, is extremely sensitive to **stress and toxins** such as halogens, toxic metals, drugs etc., which interfere with the synthesis, transport, and utilization of T-4 (thyroxine) and T-3 (triiodothyronine).

- Thyroiditis is the most common thyroid condition, leading to either hypothyroidism (Hashimoto's and sub-acute thyroiditis) or hyperthyroidism (Grave's disease). Hypothyroidism due to thyroiditis is the most common. Thyroiditis can present with normal, elevated, or decreased levels of thyroid hormone at any time.

- Functional chemistry analysis for thyroid status should consist of TSH, T-3, T-4, T-3 uptake, and free T-3 & T-4 levels. In our opinion these are the most useful tests to order.

- Multiple tests found on a thyroid panel taken independently are often misleading and inadequate in determining thyroid status. TSH, FTI, T-3 uptake, T-3, T-4, Free T-3 and T-4 are best analyzed collectively with attention to specific patterns.

- FTI (Free thyroxine Index) is a test that is often included in thyroid panels. It is an estimate calculated from total T-4 and T-3 uptake. It is usually proportional to actual free T-4 but is an imperfect measurement as it is quite possible to obtain a normal FTI with an abnormal T-3 uptake or T-4. An increased FTI is usually associated with hyperthyroidism, while a low level is associated with hypothyroidism. Although a part of many panels, this test is **not** recommended as it has been replaced by more accurate tests, such as free T-3 or thyroxine-binding globulin.

T-3

Background

T-3 is the most active thyroid hormone and is primarily produced from the conversion of thyroxine (T-4) in the peripheral tissue. T-3 has three iodine atoms attached to the tyrosine molecule as compared to the 4 iodine atoms in T-4. Approximately one-third of T-4 is converted to T-3. T-3 is more metabolically active than T-4 and its systemic effects are shorter. T-3 will bind to protein (thyroxine-binding globulin, transthyretin, albumin) less efficiently and for a shorter duration than T-4.

Discussion

Measuring total T-3 can be very useful in the diagnosis of Hyperthyroidism and Thyrotoxicosis. However, it is of limited value independently in the diagnosis of Hypothyroidism.

T-3 exists in two forms in the serum. The majority of T-3 is bound to protein and less than 1% of the total T-3 is unbound. Unbound T-3 is known as Free T-3.

Free T-3 (FT-3)

Most labs routinely measure total circulating T-3, which is largely protein-bound but not necessarily available for metabolic activity. Free T-3 is more available for tissue receptors and provides a more accurate measurement for thyroid assessment.

Ranges:

	Standard U.S. Units	Standard International Units
Conventional Laboratory Range	80 – 230 ng/dL	1.23 – 3.53 nmol/L
Optimal Range	100 – 230 ng/dL	1.54 – 3.53 nmol/L
Alarm Ranges	< 70 or > 230 ng/dL	< 1.07 or > 3.53 nmol/L

When would you run this test?

1. T-3 is useful in the diagnosis of thyroid disorders

Clinical implications

HIGH

Clinical Implication	Additional information
Hyperthyroidism	Although less common than hypothyroidism, the following pattern may help elucidate a developing or existent hyperthyroid state. **Pattern:** If T-3 is increased (>230 or 3.53 nmol/L) with decreased TSH (<2.0) and increased T-3 uptake (>37), FTI, and/or T-4 (>12 or 154.4 nmol/L) then hyperthyroidism is **probable**. Consider running thyroid antibody studies to rule out Hashimoto's thyroiditis and Grave's disease. **Please see the special topic on page 176 for more details.** Rule out food allergy/sensitivities, environmental sensitivities, recent immunizations/inoculations, viral infections, and other auto-immune problems in any cases of suspected hyperthyroidism. Some of the clinical signs of hyperthyroidism include: 1. Difficulty gaining weight, even with large appetite 2. Nervous, emotional, can't work under pressure 3. Inward trembling 4. Flush easily 5. Fast pulse at rest 6. Intolerance to high temperatures
Iodine deficiency	Although thought of as rare, iodine deficiency is actually quite common as there are many reasons for its deficiency. A poor diet and exposure to many halogen compounds can interfere with iodine metabolism (i.e. chlorine, bromine, fluoride). These common compounds render normal iodine uptake extremely difficult and may displace normal stores. **Please see the special topic on functional tests for hypothyroidism on page 176 for more details.**

	Pattern: If T-3 is increased (>230 or 3.53 nmol/L) along with a decreased T-4 (<6 or 7.2 nmol/L) and T-3-uptake (<27) and a usually normal or mildly elevated TSH (>4.4), then suspect an iodine deficiency.
Other conditions associated with ↑ T-3 levels include	Protein malnutrition Renal disease Liver disease

LOW

Clinical Implication	Additional information
Primary hypothyroidism	With a decreased T-3 level (<100 or 1.54 nmol/L) there is an increased association with clinical hypothyroidism. It cannot be used to make a diagnosis of hypothyroidism. However, some reports suggest that occasionally persons have mildly hypothyroid T-4 levels but enough T-3 secretion by the thyroid to maintain a clinically functional thyroid state.
Selenium deficiency	If the T-3 is reduced (<100 or 1.54 nmol/L) or T-3 uptake (<27) is reduced along with a normal TSH and T-4 level, consider Selenium deficiency. Inactive T-4 is converted into T-3, the active thyroid hormone, by cleaving an iodine molecule from its structure. Selenium plays an active role in this cleaving process.
Other conditions associated with decreased T-3 levels include	Pregnancy Prescribed drug or radiation therapy for hyperthyroidism Severe liver disease

Adrenal-Thyroid relationship

Increased levels of the stress hormone cortisol, produced in the adrenal cortex, frequently results in production of an inactive form of T-3 (reverse T-3). Reverse T-3 binds to thyroid hormone receptors on the cells causing an increase in tissue resistance to T-3. Serum T-3 and T-3 uptake will often be normal coupled with symptoms and physical findings of thyroid hypofunction. T-3 (triiodothyronine) supplementation may be helpful in ameliorating the patient's subjective complaints, but the correction for the problem should be oriented towards correcting the underlying adrenal dysfunction and normalizing the cortisol rhythm.

Interfering Factors:

Only measuring total T-3 has a few drawbacks. The first of which is that serum T-3 is affected by alterations in thyroxine-binding proteins which can alter true levels.

Falsely increased levels	Falsely decreased levels
• Following desiccated thyroid medications (several hours)	• Severe illness

Related Tests:

Serum T-3 uptake, thyroxine (T-4), free thyroxine index (FTI), thyroid stimulating hormone (TSH), thyroid binding globulin (TBG), serum triglycerides, serum cholesterol, serum calcium, serum phosphorous, RBC magnesium, serum albumin, HCT, HGB

Total T-4

Background

The major hormone secreted by the thyroid gland is thyroxine or T-4. T-4 production and secretion from the thyroid gland is stimulated by TSH. T-4 is composed of a tyrosine molecule with 4 iodine atoms attached to it, hence the name T-4. T-4 is metabolized into the active thyroid hormone T-3 (Triiodothyronine) by having an iodine molecule cleaved from the quaternary form. The majority of T-4 is transported through the blood bound to thyroxine-binding globulin (TBG), pre-albumin, and albumin.

Discussion

 T-4 conversion into T-3 is dependent upon the presence of iodine, selenium, and tyrosine amongst other nutrients. Therefore, these key nutrient deficiencies should be ruled out before instituting conventional thyroid treatment.

- Thyroxine or T-4 has wide-ranging metabolic activities in the body:
    - Basal Metabolic Rate
    - Normal growth and development
    - Metabolism of fats and proteins
    - Regulation of stress hormones and neurotransmitters
    - Immune resistance.

Free T-4 (FT-4)

Most labs routinely measure <u>total</u> circulating T-4, which is largely protein-bound but not necessarily available for metabolic activity. Free T-4 is more available for tissue receptors and provides a more accurate measurement for thyroid assessment.

Ranges:

	Standard U.S. Units	Standard International Units
Conventional Laboratory Range	4.8 – 13.2 mcg/dL	61.8 – 169.9 nmol/L
Optimal Range	6.0 – 12.0 mcg/dL	77.2 – 154.4 nmol/L
Alarm Ranges	< 5.0 or > 13.0 mcg/dL	< 65 or > 167 nmol/L

When would you run this test?

1. A test commonly used to rule-out hyperthyroidism and hypothyroidism

2. To establish maintenance doses of thyroid hormone in the treatment of hypothyroidism

Clinical implications

HIGH

Clinical Implication	Additional information
Hyperthyroidism	Although less common than hypothyroidism, the following pattern may help elucidate a developing or existent hyperthyroid state.
	Pattern:
	If T-4 is increased (>12 or 154.4 nmol/L) with a decreased TSH (<2.0) and increased T-3 (>230 or 3.53 nmol/L), FTI, and/or T-3 uptake (>37) then hyperthyroidism is **probable**. Consider running thyroid antibody studies to rule out Hashimoto's thyroiditis and Grave's disease. **Please see the special topic on page 176 for more details.**
	Rule-out food allergy/sensitivities, environmental sensitivities, recent immunizations/inoculations, viral infections, and other auto-immune problems in any cases of suspected hyperthyroidism. Some of the clinical signs of hyperthyroidism include:
	1. Difficulty gaining weight, even with large appetite
	2. Nervous, emotional, can't work under pressure
	3. Inward trembling
	4. Flush easily
	5. Fast pulse at rest
	6. Intolerance to high temperatures

Thyroid Hormone Replacement	T-4 will usually be increased (>12 or 154.4 nmol/L) along with an increased T-3 uptake (>37) with the use of synthetic thyroxine (Synthroid, Eltroxin, Levothroid, Levoxine, Levoxyl and Levo-T) and desiccated thyroid preparations (Armour thyroid, Westhroid, Thyroid strong, S-P-T, Thyrar.)	
Drug causes of ↑	❋ Oral contraceptives ❋ Exogenous estrogen use ❋ Contrast radiopaque substances used for x-ray	❋ Heroin and Methadone ❋ Propranalol
Other conditions associated with increased T-4 levels include	❋ Liver disease (cirrhosis) 🫘 Elevated metabolic activity	🫘 Pregnancy ❋ Adrenal fatigue

Wilson's Syndrome

Wilson's syndrome is a condition of abnormal conversion of T-4 into the more active T-3 in the peripheral tissue. Significant amounts of the T-4 get converted into reverse T-3, an almost biologically inactive molecule, which interferes with thyroid binding at the tissue level. Not unlike Type II diabetes, Wilson's syndrome is a problem of tissue resistance as opposed to organ dysfunction. The thyroid gland in Wilson's syndrome is usually functioning normally. In many cases the thyroid hormone tests, such as TSH are normal. There may be an associated low normal or decreased total T-3 and T-4 level and an increased reverse T-3 level.

Many types of stressors (i.e. starvation diets, pregnancy, environmental pollutants, emotional stress, and multiple drugs) can impair the peripheral conversion of T-4 to T-3.

LOW

Clinical Implication	Additional information
Primary hypothyroidism	Hypothyroidism is a very common and often undiagnosed condition. Individual blood indices are notoriously insensitive to mild or borderline cases of primary hypothyroidism. In many cases TSH levels may be within normal limits yet the patient is suffering from all the classic signs and symptoms of low thyroid. In these cases it is often more efficacious to look at more functional criteria such as basal body temperature, Achilles return reflex, and iodine status, along with history,

	other blood indices, and clinical signs and symptoms. **Please see the special topic on functional tests for hypothyroidism on page 176 for more details.** **Pattern:** If T-4 is decreased (<6 or 7.2 nmol/L) with an increased TSH (> 4.4 µIU/ml), a normal or decreased T-3 uptake (<27) and/or T-3 level (<100 or 1.54 nmol/L), and an increased cholesterol (>220 or 5.69 mmol/L) and triglyceride level (>110 or 1.24 mmol/L), primary hypothyroidism is **probable**. Some of the clinical signs of hypothyroidism include: 1. Difficulty losing weight 2. Mentally sluggish, reduced initiative 3. Easily fatigued, sleepy during the day 4. Sensitive to cold, poor circulation (cold hands and feet) 5. Constipation, chronic 6. Excessive hair loss and / or coarse hair 7. Morning headaches, wear off during the day 8. Loss of lateral 1/3 of eyebrow 9. Seasonal sadness
Iodine deficiency	Although thought of as rare, iodine deficiency is actually quite common as there are many reasons for its deficiency. A poor diet and exposure to many halogen compounds can interfere with iodine metabolism (i.e. chlorine, bromine, fluoride). These common compounds render normal iodine uptake extremely difficult and may displace normal stores. **Please see the special topic on functional tests for hypothyroidism on page 176 for more details on iodine testing.** **Pattern:** If T-4 is decreased (<6 or 7.2 nmol/L) along with a decreased T-3-uptake (<27), an increased T-3 (>230 or 3.53 nmol/L) and a usually normal or mildly elevated TSH (>4.4), then suspect an iodine deficiency.
Steroid Usage	The use of anabolic steroids should be ruled-out when the T-4 level is decreased along with an increased T-3-uptake.

Drug causes of ↓	✳ Exogenous androgens	✳ Exogenous T-3
	✳ Anti-convulsants	✳ Anti-coagulants
	✳ Salicylates	
Other conditions associated with decreased T-4 levels include	✳ Chronic liver disease 🌰 Protein malnutrition	✳ Nephrosis

Interfering Factors:

Falsely increased levels	Falsely decreased levels
• Pregnancy- especially 2nd and 3rd trimester due to increased estrogen levels • Thyroid treatment within one month of testing	• None noted

Related Tests:

Serum T-3 uptake, T-3, free thyroxine index (FTI), thyroid stimulating hormone (TSH), thyroid binding globulin (TBG), serum triglycerides, serum cholesterol, serum calcium, serum phosphorous, RBC magnesium, serum albumin, HCT, HGB

T-3 Uptake

Background

The T-3 uptake test has nothing to do with actual T-3 levels, as the name might suggest, instead it is an indirect measurement of the unsaturated binding sites on the thyroxine-binding proteins (thyroid binding globulin, transthyretin, and albumin). This test should only be ordered as part of a thyroid panel including T-4 and is also used in the calculation of Free Thyroxine Index (FTI).

Discussion

 T-3 uptake is dependent on the number of binding sites on the thyroxine-binding protein, any changes in the amount of thyroxine-binding proteins will affect the T-3 uptake. Thyroxine-binding globulin abnormalities may be congenital, drug induced or caused by non-thyroid related illnesses such as liver and kidney disease. Any conditions or situations that decrease thyroxine-binding globulins will increase the T-3 uptake, and vice versa.

• The T-3 uptake can be helpful to rule-out a laboratory error in T-4 increase. A true T-4 increase can be confirmed if both the T-3 uptake and the T-4 levels are increased.

Ranges:

	Standard U.S. Units	**Standard International Units**
Conventional Laboratory Range	22 – 39% of uptake	22 – 39% of uptake
Optimal Range	27 – 37% of uptake	27 – 37% of uptake
Alarm Ranges	< 20% or > 39%	< 20% or > 39%

When would you run this test?

1. This test should be run as part of a complete thyroid panel. It is not helpful to run this test by itself.

2. This test can help rule-out laboratory error as a cause of T-4 increase.

<u>Clinical implications</u>

HIGH

Clinical Implication	Additional information
Hyperthyroidism	Although less common than hypothyroidism, the following pattern may help elucidate a developing or existent hyperthyroid state.
	<u>Pattern:</u>
	If T-3 uptake is increased (>37) with a decreased TSH (2.0) and increased T-3 (>230 or 3.53 nmol/L), FTI, and/or T-4 (>12 or 154.4 nmol/L) then hyperthyroidism is **probable**. Consider running thyroid antibody studies to rule out Hashimoto's thyroiditis and Grave's disease. **Please see the special topic on page 178 for more details.**
	Rule out food allergy/sensitivities, environmental sensitivities, recent immunizations/inoculations, viral infections, and other auto-immune problems in any cases of suspected hyperthyroidism. Some of the clinical signs of hyperthyroidism include:
	1. Difficulty gaining weight, even with large appetite
	2. Nervous, emotional, can't work under pressure
	3. Inward trembling
	4. Flush easily
	5. Fast pulse at rest
	6. Intolerance to high temperatures
Thyroid Hormone Replacement	T-3 uptake will usually be increased (>37) with the use of synthetic thyroxine (Synthroid, Eltroxin, Levothroid, Levoxine, Levoxyl, and Levo-T) and desiccated thyroid preparations (Armour thyroid, Westhroid, Thyroid strong, S-P-T, Thyrar.)
Drug causes of ⬆	✳ Exogenous androgens ✳ Dicumerol ✳ Heparin ✳ Anabolic steroids ✳ Salicylates (large-doses)	✳ Drugs that compete with a T-3 and T-4 binding-sites on thyroxine-binding globulin or albumin: Phenytoin, Valproic acid, and Ponstel
Other conditions associated with increased T-3 uptake levels include	⬤ Protein malnutrition ⬤ Acute stress	✳ Renal disease ✳ Liver disease

LOW

Clinical Implication	Additional information
Primary hypothyroidism	Hypothyroidism is a very common and often undiagnosed condition. Individual blood indices are notoriously insensitive to mild or borderline cases of primary hypothyroidism. In many cases TSH levels may be within normal limits yet the patient is suffering from all the classic signs and symptoms of low thyroid. In these cases it is often more efficacious to look at more functional criteria such as basal body temperature, Achilles return reflex, and iodine status, along with history, other blood indices, and clinical signs and symptoms.
	Please see the special topic on functional tests for hypothyroidism on page 176 for more details.
	<u>**Pattern:**</u>
	If T-3 uptake is decreased (<27) with an increased TSH (> 4.4), a normal or decreased T-4 (<6 or 7.2 nmol/L) and/or T-3 level (< 100 or 1.54 nmol/L), and an increased cholesterol (>220 or 5.69 mmol/L) and triglyceride level (>110 or 1.24 mmol/L), primary hypothyroidism is **probable**.
	Some of the clinical signs of hypothyroidism include:
	1. Difficulty losing weight
	2. Mentally sluggish, reduced initiative
	3. Easily fatigued, sleepy during the day
	4. Sensitive to cold, poor circulation (cold hands and feet)
	5. Constipation, chronic
	6. Excessive hair loss and / or coarse hair
	7. Morning headaches, wear off during the day
	8. Loss of lateral 1/3 of eyebrow
	9. Seasonal sadness
Secondary Hypothyroidism **(Anterior Pituitary Hypofunction)**	Thyroid hypofunction is often secondary to an anterior pituitary hypofunction (Secondary Hypothyroidism). If the subjective indications of thyroid hypofunction are present and a decreased T-3 uptake (<27) and normal T-4, T-3 and FTI, with the TSH <2.0, **Anterior Pituitary Hypofunction** should be considered.
	If serum triglycerides are elevated (>110 or 1.24 mmol/L) and the total cholesterol levels are decreased (<150 or 3.9 mmol/L), then secondary hypothyroidism is **probable**.
	Anterior pituitary hypofunction is a common problem and one

	that is frequently mistaken for thyroid hypofunction (the subjective indications are usually identical and the patient's axillary temperature will frequently be below normal). Some of the common clinical indications of an anterior pituitary dysfunction include: 1. Decreased libido 2. Weight gain around hips or waist 3. Menstrual irregularities 4. Delayed sexual development (after age 13) 5. Unresponsive thyroid treatment 6. Hypoglycemia due to concomitant adrenal insufficiency
Selenium deficiency	If the T-3 uptake is reduced (<27) or T-3 is reduced (<100 or 1.54 nmol/L) along with a normal TSH and T-4 level, consider Selenium deficiency. Inactive T-4 is converted into T-3, the active thyroid hormone via the activity of the deiodinase enzyme. Selenium plays an active role in this process by cleaving an iodine molecule from the T-4 molecule.
Iodine deficiency	Although thought of as rare, iodine deficiency is actually quite common as there are many reasons for its deficiency. A poor diet and exposure to many halogen compounds can interfere with iodine metabolism (i.e. chlorine, bromine, fluoride). These common compounds render normal iodine uptake extremely difficult and may displace normal stores. **Please see the special topic on functional tests for hypothyroidism on page 176 for more details on iodine testing.** **Pattern:** If T-3 uptake is decreased (<27) along with a decreased T-4 (<6 or 7.2 nmol/L) and an increased T-3 (>230 or 3.53 nmol/L) and a usually normal or mildly elevated TSH (>4.4), then suspect an iodine deficiency.

Drug causes of ↓	❋ Oral contraceptives ❋ Exogenous estrogen ❋ Perphrenazine (Trilafon)	❋ Heroin and Methadone (occasionally) ❋ Anovulatory drugs
Other conditions associated with decreased T-3 uptake	❋ Pregnancy ❋ Severe liver disease	❋ Prescribed drug or radiation therapy for hyperthyroidism

Interfering Factors:

Falsely increased levels	Falsely decreased levels
• None noted	• None noted

Related Tests:

Serum T-3, thyroxine (T-4), free thyroxine index (FTI), thyroid stimulating hormone (TSH), thyroid binding globulin (TBG), serum triglycerides, serum cholesterol, serum calcium, serum phosphorous, RBC magnesium, serum albumin, HCT, HGB.

Erythrocyte Sedimentation Rate

Background

Sedimentation occurs when the erythrocytes clump or aggregate together. The ESR is the rate at which erythrocytes settle out of anti-coagulated blood in 1 hour. The ESR is useful for determining the level of tissue destruction, inflammation, and is an indication that a disease process is ongoing and must be investigated.

Discussion

 The test is based on the fact that certain blood proteins will become altered in inflammatory conditions, causing aggregation of the red blood cells. Aggregation causes the cells to become heavier and fall more rapidly when placed in a special vertical test tube. The faster the sedimentation, the higher the ESR. Increased albumin levels in the blood will affect sedimentation by causing a decreased ESR. Albumin is produced in the liver, therefore liver dysfunction can cause a decreased albumin production, which may increase the ESR.

Ranges: Using the Westergren method

	Standard U.S. Units	**Standard International Units**
Conventional Laboratory Range	**Males**: 0-15 mm/hour **Females**: 0-20 mm/hour	**Males**: 0-15 mm/hour **Females**: 0-20 mm/hour
Optimal Range	**Males**: <5 mm/hour **Females**: <10 mm/hour	**Males**: <5 mm/hour **Females**: <10 mm/hour
Alarm Ranges	**Males**: >45 mm/hour **Females**: >45 mm/hour	**Males**: >45 mm/hour **Females**: >45 mm/hour

When would you run this test?

1. To determine the level of inflammation or destruction with any disease process.

2. To follow the course of an established condition increasing as the condition gets worse and decreasing as the condition abates.

Clinical implications

HIGH

Clinical Implication	Additional information	
Tissue inflammation	Any type of inflammation in the body will cause an increased ESR. As a generalized indicator of inflammation, an ESR will be increased in most cases of tissue inflammation (SLE, RA, gout, arthritis, nephritis, nephrosis, endocarditis).	
Tissue destruction	An increased ESR is seen in carcinoma, lymphoma, and neoplasms as well as any process that involves cell or tissue destruction e.g. auto-immune processes.	
Musculoskeletal conditions	• In rheumatic, gonorrheal, and acute gouty arthritis the rate is greatly increased. • In osteoarthritis the rate is slightly increased.	
Cardiovascular conditions	• In myocardial infarction, the rate is increased • In angina pectoris the rate is not increased	
Malignant diseases	In multiple myeloma, lymphoma, and metastatic cancer, the rate is very high. The degree of elevation does not correspond with prognosis	
Other conditions associated with increased ESR levels include	✳ Uncomplicated viral disease ✳ Active renal failure with heart failure	✳ Active allergy ✳ Peptic ulcer ✳ Infectious mononucleosis

Interfering Factors:

Anemia will invalidate the ESR results.

The sed. rate may be very high in apparently healthy women over the age of 70

Falsely increased levels	Falsely decreased levels
• Presence of fibrinogen, globulins and cholesterol • Pregnancy after 12 weeks until 4th week postpartum • Young children • Menstruation • Certain drugs: heparin and oral contraceptives • High hemoglobin values	• Having blood sample stand for more than 24 hours • High blood sugar • High albumin levels • High phospholipid levels • Certain drugs: steroids, high dose aspirin

<u>Related Tests:</u>

C-Reactive Protein, serum protein electrophoresis (SPE), WBC with differential, RBC and indices, albumin, total protein, ALP and the isoenzymes of ALP (liver, bone and intestine), ANA, Rheumatoid factors, fibrinogen.

COMPLETE BLOOD COUNT

White Blood Cell count

Background

White blood cells or leukocytes of the peripheral blood are divided into 2 groups:

1. Granulocytes:

This group consists of neutrophils, basophils, and eosinophils, which are formed in the bone marrow and receives their name from the granules that are present in the cytoplasm. They also contain a multi-lobed nucleus and are often referred to as "polys" or polymorphonuclear leukocytes (PMNs).

2. Agranulocytes:

This group consists of monocytes and lymphocytes. They have no granules in their cytoplasm and non-lobular nuclei. Monocytes originate in the bone marrow, and lymphocytes are formed from lymphoblasts in the reticuloendothelial tissues of the spleen, lymph glands, tonsils, thymus, and appendix.

Discussion

 The number of leukocytes in the blood is regulated by the endocrine system. Production from the blood-forming organs, their storage, release from the tissue, and ultimate disintegration is affected by hormones. The lifespan of leukocytes varies from 13 to 20 days.

- Leukocytes fight infection, defend the body via phagocytosis, and produce, transport and distribute antibodies as part of the immune process.

- It is important to look at the WBC differential to locate the source of an increased or decreased WBC count.

Ranges: The following ranges are expressed as a % of the total WBC count

	Standard U.S. Units	Standard International Units
Conventional Laboratory Range	$3.7 - 11.0 \times 10^3/mm^3$	$3.7 - 11.0 \times 10^9/L$
Optimal Range	$5.0 - 7.5 \times 10^3/mm^3$	$5.0 - 7.5 \times 10^9/L$
Alarm Ranges	< 3.0 or $> 13.0 \times 10^3/mm^3$	< 3.0 or $> 13.0 \times 10^9/L$

When would you run this test?

1. To screen the body's ability to respond to infection and inflammation.

Clinical implications

HIGH (Leukocytosis)

Clinical Implication	Additional information
Childhood diseases (Measles, Mumps, Chicken-pox, Rubella, etc.)	Total WBC is increased early (>7.5) in the disease process and will be decreased later (<5.0). The increase in total WBC may be so great as to suggest leukemia. Such a leukocytosis of a temporary nature must be distinguished from leukemia. In general the following common patterns may be seen in childhood disease: **Neutrophils**: Increased early (>60). Decreased later (<40) **Lymphocytes**: Decreased early (<24) . Increased later (>44) The findings relative to the WBC differential are variable due to the increases or decreases in the other WBC fractions (eosinophils, Monocytes, basophils)
Acute viral infection	This is a strong inflammatory process so expect to see an increased ESR. The total WBC will be elevated (>7.5) due to the increased levels of individual fractions. Increased Lymphocytes (>44) and normal Neutrophils = Acute viral picture Increased Monocytes (>7) indicate the recovery period. Increased Bands- Expect to see increased Band cells in the acute phase as the body is pumping out immature neutrophils to cope with the infection. Bands can be used to help differentiate an active from a chronic infection. In the active phase of infection bands will tend to become increased and their levels tend to normalize during recovery or during the chronic phase. Checking viral titers may be helpful
Acute bacterial infection	This is a strong inflammatory process so expect to see an increased ESR. The total WBC will be elevated (>7.5) due to the increased levels of individual fractions. Increased Neutrophils (>60) and normal Lymphocytes = Acute bacterial picture

	Increased Monocytes (>7) indicate the recovery period.
	Increased Bands- Expect to see increased Band cells in the acute phase as the body is pumping out immature neutrophils to cope with the infection. Bands can be used to help differentiate an active from a chronic infection. In the active phase of infection bands will tend to become increased and their levels tend to normalize during recovery or during the chronic phase.
Stressful situations	Any stressful situation, which leads to an increase in epinephrine production, may cause an increase in the total WBC (>7.5).
Highly refined diets	The total WBC may be slightly above the optimum level for people on a diet of highly refined foods
Other conditions associated with increased WBC levels include	Intestinal parasites Free radical pathology (neoplasm) Adrenal dysfunction Late pregnancy Asthma Emphysema Polycythemia Influenza with secondary bacterial infection

LOW (Leukopenia)

Clinical Implication	Additional information
Chronic viral infection	In a chronic viral infection the total WBC count will be decreased (<5.5), as the body is using up its WBCs. **Pattern:** Decreased total WBC (<5.5), increased lymphocyte count (>44), decreased neutrophils (<40), decreased LDH isoenzymes due to a decrease in the total WBC and an increased monocytes (>7) during the recovery phase.
Chronic bacterial infection	The total WBC count in a chronic bacterial infection will often be opposite of that seen with active infection: **Pattern:** Decreased total WBC (<5.5), increased neutrophils (>60), decreased lymphocyte count (<24), and decreased LDH isoenzymes due to a decrease in the total WBC. Expect to see an increased monocyte count (>7) during the recovery phase.

Pancreatic insufficiency	The body responds to pancreatic insufficiency by using phagocytic white cells to do the job of breaking down food and clearing food residue from the system. This is known as leukocytic auto digestion and can cause a decreased white count (<5.5).
Systemic Lupus Erythematosis (SLE)	SLE is a disease characterized by inflammation in several organ systems and the production of auto-antibodies that cause cellular injury. It is a disease of extreme variability in clinical and laboratory presentation. Nearly half of all people suffering from SLE have leukopenia, and anemia is usually present in the active disease. **Pattern**: SLE is **possible** with decreased WBC count (<5.5) and C-complement, and an increased ANA, Alpha 1 globulin, C reactive protein, and gamma globulin.
Decreased production	If the following chemistries are out of range we can suspect a functional decreased production from the bone marrow: **Pattern:** Decreased total WBC (<5.5), RBCs (<3.9 in women or 4.2 in men), cholesterol (<150 or 3.9 mmol/L), magnesium, and BUN (<10 or 3.57 mmol/L) with an increased MCV (>89.9). Certain drugs, chemotherapeutic agents, radiation, and heavy metals can cause bone marrow depression.
Raw food diet	The total WBC (<5.5) will frequently be slightly below the optimum range for patients on a diet high in raw foods.
Other conditions associated with decreased WBC levels include	* Hepatitis * Free radical diseases (neoplasm) * Vitamin B-12, vitamin B-6, and folic acid anemia * Anterior pituitary dysfunction * Adrenal dysfunction * Parathyroid hyperfunction * Intestinal parasites (chronic) * Rheumatoid arthritis * Multiple food allergies.

Interfering Factors:

- **Hourly rhythm**: There is an early morning low and a late afternoon peak

- **Age**: In newborns and infants the count is high and gradually tapers in children until adult levels are reached at about 21.

- Hormonal influences in females over the age of 40 may cause a lower than normal total WBC count.

- An increase may be seen when there is a large number of nucleated RBCs

Related Tests:

A significantly increased or decreased total WBC is justification to conduct further immune testing (T and B lymphocyte subset assay, immunoglobulins, C-Reactive Protein, etc.)

Red Blood Cell Count

Discussion

The red blood cell functions to carry oxygen from the lungs to the body tissues and to transfer carbon dioxide from the tissues to the lungs. To enable the maximum amount of hemoglobin to be used, the red cell is shaped like a biconcave disk, affording an increased surface area. The cell is able to change its shape when necessary to allow its passage through smaller capillaries.

This test determines the total number of cells or erythrocytes found in a cubic millimeter of blood.

Ranges:

	Standard U.S. Units	Standard International Units
Conventional Laboratory Range	**Males**: $4.6 - 6.0 \times 10^6 /mm^3$	**Males**: $4.6 - 6.0 \times 10^{12} /L$
	Females: $3.8 - 5.1$	**Females**: $3.8 - 5.1$
Optimal Range	**Males**: $4.2 - 4.9 \times 10^6 /mm^3$	**Males**: $4.2 - 4.9 \times 10^{12} /L$
	Females: $4.0 - 4.5$	**Females**: $4.0 - 4.5$
Alarm Ranges	**Males**: <3.8 or >6.0	**Males**: <3.8 or >6.0
	Females:<3.5 or >5.0	**Females**:<3.5 or >5.0

When would you run this test?

1. To evaluate anemia: The red blood cell count is an important measurement when evaluating anemia. The RBC count should be evaluated with HCT, HGB, RBC, MCV, MCH, serum ferritin, serum iron and TIBC or % transferrin saturation to determine the cause of anemia and the type of anemia.

2. To screen for dehydration

Clinical implications

HIGH

Clinical Implication	Additional information
Relative increases in RBC count	Whenever there is a decrease in blood volume, you will see a relative increase in the RBC count (>4.5 in women and >4.9 in men) usually with an increased HCT (>44 or 0.44 in women and >48 or 0.48 in men), and HGB (>14.5 or 145 in women or 15 or 150 in men).
	Common causes of a relative increase in RBC count include:
	• Dehydration- decreased fluid intake, vomiting, diarrhea
	• Stress
	• Tobacco use
	• Overuse of diuretics
Dehydration	If the RBC count is increased suspect dehydration. Dehydration is a very common problem and should be factored into your blood chemistry and CBC analysis. **Please see special topic on page 90 for more details.**
	Pattern:
	Suspect a short-term (acute) dehydration if there is an increased HGB (>14.5 or 145 in women or 15 or 150 in men) and/or HCT (>44 or 0.44 in women and >48 or 0.48 in men) along with an increased RBC count (>4.5 in women and >4.9 in men). A relative increase in Sodium (>142) and Potassium (>4.5) can be noted as well.
	Suspect a long-term (chronic) dehydration if any of the above findings are accompanied by an increased Albumin (>5.0 or 50 g/L), increased BUN (>16 or 5.71 mmol/L), and/or serum Protein (7.4 or 74 g/L).
Respiratory distress	In severe cases of asthma and emphysema you can expect an increased red cell count with decreased HGB (<13.5 or 135 g/L in women and <14 or 140 in men) and HCT (<37 or 0.37 in women and 40 or 0.4 in men). The body responds to an inability to fully oxygenate the blood with an increase in red blood cells.
Vitamin C need	An increased RBC level is associated with vitamin C need.
	Pattern:
	Albumin will frequently be decreased (<4.0 or 40g/L) along

	a decreased HCT (<37 or 0.37 in women and 40 or 0.4 in men), HGB (<13.5 or 135 g/L in women and <14 or 140 in men), MCH (28), MCHC (<32), serum iron (< 50 or 8.96 μmol/dL). There will also be an increased MCV (>90), alkaline phosphatase (>100), and fibrinogen.
	Both the lingual ascorbic acid test and Urinary vitamin C will generally be out of range. **Please see the special topic on the lingual ascorbic acid test on page 218 for details.**
Polycythemia vera	A myeloproliferative disease that causes an increase in all blood cell lines. This disease will cause an increased HCT (<37 or 0.37 in women and 40 or 0.4 in men), HGB (<13.5 or 135 g/L in women and <14 or 140 in men), total bilirubin (>1.2 or 20.5 μmol/dL), uric acid (>5.9 or > 351 μmol/dL), basophils (>1), and ALP (>100). Further testing with blood coagulation studies is needed
Drug causes of ↑	※ Gentamicin ※ Methyldopa
Other conditions associated with increased RBC levels include	Adrenal hyperfunction ※ Cystic fibrosis

LOW

Clinical Implication	Additional information
Anemia	A condition in which there is a decreased amount of hemoglobin, a decreased number of circulating RBCs, and a decrease in the hematocrit. Anemia is a <u>symptom</u> not a disease, and the cause of an anemia must be sought out: • Deficiencies of iron and certain vitamins (B12, folate, B6, C) and copper • Blood loss • Increased destruction The following are some of the different nutritional types of anemia.
Anemia- Iron deficiency	This is the most prevalent anemia worldwide. The major causes are: 1. Dietary inadequacies

2. Malabsorption

3. Increased iron loss

4. Increased iron requirements

Pattern:

 If there is a decreased HCT (<37 or 0.37 in women and 40 or 0.4 in men) and/or HGB (<13.5 or 135 g/L in women and <14 or 140 in men), MCH (<28), MCV (<82), and MCHC (<32), and a decreased serum iron (< 50 or 8.96 µmol/dL), ferritin (<33 in men and 10 in women), % transferrin saturation, and an increased RDW (>13), then iron anemia is **probable**.

If TIBC is increased (>350 or 62.7 µmol/dL), internal/microscopic bleeding is **possible**, and should be ruled out with reticulocyte count, urinalysis, and/or stool analysis.

Iron deficiency anemia may be secondary to hypochlorhydria if serum phosphorous is decreased (<3.0 or 0.97 mmol/L) and serum globulin is increased (>2.8 or 28 g/L) or decreased (<2.4 or 24 g/L).

Some of the subjective indicators for iron need are:

1. Prolonged fatigue, particularly in pregnancy

2. Blue sclera of the eyes

3. Pica and a desire to chew ice

4. Inability to tolerate cold

Anemia- B12/folic acid	**Pattern:**
	If there is decreased RBCs (<3.9 in women or 4.2 in men) with a decreased HCT (<37 or 0.37 in women and 40 or 0.4 in men) and/or HGB (<13.5 or 135 g/L in women and <14 or 140 in men), and uric acid (<3.5 or 208 µmol/dL) and an increased MCH (>31.9), MCV (>90), RDW (>13), LDH (>200) (especially the LDH-1 isoenzyme fraction) and serum iron (>100 or 17.91 µmol/dL), then B12/folic acid anemia is **probable**.
	Often you will see decreased WBC (<5.0) and neutrophils (<40) and an increased LDH (>200) in megaloblastic anemia (i.e. anemia of large cells). Check with methylmalonic acid and homocysteine.

	The presence of hypersegmented neutrophils (5 or more lobes in more than 5% of all neutrophils) has been reported to be more sensitive and reliable than an elevated MCV in detecting megaloblastic anemia and is not affected by coexisting iron deficiency. If MCV is >97 oral supplementation may be ineffective. B12 injections may be needed.
Anemia- Copper	If there is decreased RBCs (<3.9 in women or 4.2 in men) with a decreased HCT (<37 or 0.37 in women and 40 or 0.4 in men) and/or HGB (<13.5 or 135 g/L in women and <14 or 140 in men) , and low high MCV (>89.9), an increased to normal MCH (>31.9), and an increased or decreased hair copper, then copper anemia is **possible**. Check serum or WBC copper.
Internal bleeding	An unrecognized internal bleed can cause a gradual decrease in RBCs due to the loss of blood. Check reticulocyte count. Internal bleeding is a serious condition and should be referred to a specialist qualified to diagnose and treat this condition.

Other conditions associated with decreased RBC levels include	🍂 Vitamin B-6 🍂 Liver dysfunction ✳ Renal dysfunction	✳ Hereditary anemia 🍂 Free radical pathology

Interfering Factors:

Age: A newborn has a higher RBC count than an adult. It then drops to the lowest point in life at 2-4 months. Normal adult levels are reached by 14 years of age. This is maintained until old age when we see a gradual decline.

Falsely increased levels	Falsely decreased levels
• **Altitude**: higher the altitude the greater the increase in RBCs • **Dehydration**: causes a concentration of the blood and may obscure anemia	• **Posture**: When blood is taken from a healthy person in the recumbent position, the RBC count is lower than normal. In a person with anemia, the count will be even lower • **Pregnancy**: the normal number of RBCs gets diluted in the increased volume of fluid • **Drugs**: many drugs can cause a decrease in RBCs

Related Tests:

HGB, HCT, MCV, MCH, serum ferritin, serum iron, TIBC or % transferrin saturation, reticulocyte count.

Reticulocyte count

Discussion

 A reticulocyte is a young, immature red blood cell. It is non-nucleated, yet contains RNA that stains a gray-blue color when stained with brilliant Cresyl blue. A red blood cell is a reticulocyte for the first 1-2 days after being released into general circulation, and before it reaches its full mature state. A small number of reticulocytes are found in circulating blood.

- The reticulocyte count must be viewed in relation to the total red blood cell count.

Ranges:

	Standard U.S. Units	Standard International Units
Conventional Laboratory Range	0.5 – 1%	0.005 – 0.01
Optimal Range	0.5 – 1%	0.005 – 0.01
Alarm Ranges	>2%	0.02

When would you run this test?

1. To help in anemia differentiation: a reticulocyte count may be used to differentiate anemias caused by bone marrow failure from those caused by blood loss or destruction.

2. To measure treatment effectiveness: The reticulocyte count is an excellent means for:

    a. Measuring the effect of therapy with microscopic internal bleeding (it will decrease if the therapy is successful).

    b. Measuring the efficacy of supplementation in cofactor anemia(s) (if the reticulocyte count is decreased, it will increase when supplementation for vitamin B-12, vitamin B-6 or folic acid anemia is successful).

3. This is an excellent test for confirming chronic microscopic bleeding.

Clinical implications

HIGH

An increased reticulocyte count indicates that an increased production of red blood cells is occurring in the bone marrow in response to premature destruction or loss.

Clinical Implication	Additional information
Presence of an occult or unknown disease e.g. microscopic internal bleeding or hemolysis	The presence of reticulocytes can lead to the recognition of an otherwise unknown or unrecognized illness e.g. a chronic microscopic bleed or unrecognized hemolysis (sickle cell disease or thalassemia).
	Pattern:
	The probability that there is a microscopic bleed somewhere in the body increases as the reticulocyte count increases. Expect to see an increased reticulocyte count (>1) with a concomitant decreased TIBC (<250 or 44.8 µmol/dL) or % transferrin saturation and a decreased serum iron (< 50 or 8.96 µmol/dL).
	Internal bleeding is a serious problem and should be handled by a doctor qualified to diagnose and treat internal bleeding.
Anemia- hemolytic	An increased reticulocyte (>1) is more often seen in hemolytic anemias where there is a large red cell destruction.
Following treatment of anemia	• An increase in reticulocytes may be used to follow effectiveness of treatment. • There is a proportional increase when treating pernicious anemia with B12 therapy.

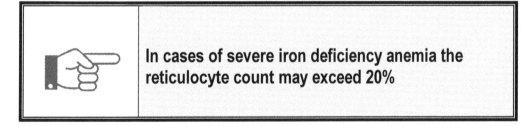

In cases of severe iron deficiency anemia the reticulocyte count may exceed 20%

Other conditions associated with increased reticulocyte levels include	Free radical pathology Hereditary anemia Vitamin C anemia	Heavy metal body burdens Renal dysfunction Liver dysfunction

LOW

A ↓ reticulocyte count means that the bone marrow is not producing enough red blood cells

Clinical Implication	Additional information
Anemia	Seen in iron deficiency anemia and aplastic anemia, where there is a persistent deficiency in red blood cells. Reticulocytes can also be seen in untreated pernicious anemia.
Other conditions associated with decreased reticulocyte levels include	Vitamin B-12, vitamin B-6 and folic acid anemia Adrenal hypofunction Anterior pituitary hypofunction

Interfering Factors:

Falsely increased levels	Falsely decreased levels
• In infants and pregnancy • The presence of Howell-Jolley bodies can falsely elevate the count	• Recently transfused patients

Related Tests:

TIBC, % transferrin saturation, serum iron, serum ferritin, HGB, HCT, RBC, MCV and MCH.

Hematocrit

Background

The hematocrit (HCT) is expressed as a percentage of the volume of red blood cells in a known volume of centrifuged blood.

Discussion

The hematocrit will usually parallel the RBC count when the cells are of a normal size. This pattern does not hold true when the RBCs are small (microcytic) or large (macrocytic).

The hematocrit should be evaluated with HGB, RBC, MCV, MCH, serum ferritin, serum iron, and TIBC (or transferrin) to determine the cause of anemia and the type of anemia.

Often patients with low normal serum iron, serum ferritin, HGB, and HCT are generally more active and healthy than those patients with high normal or increased values.

Ranges:

	Standard U.S. Units	Standard International Units
Conventional Laboratory Range	**Male**: 36 – 50%	**Male**: 0.36 – 0.50
	Female: 34 – 44%	**Female**: 0.34 – 0.44
Optimal Range	**Males**: 40 – 48%	**Males**: 0.40 – 0.48
	Females: 37 – 44%	**Females**: 0.37 – 0.44
Alarm Ranges	**Males**: <32% or >55%	**Males**: <0.32 or >0.55
	Females:<32% or >55%	**Females**:<0.32 or >0.55

When would you run this test?

1. Determining degree of anemia and polycythemia: Although it cannot differentiate the type of anemia, the hematocrit, along with RBC count and hemoglobin can help determine the degree of anemia and polycythemia.

2. Evaluating treatment of anemia: As an anemia is treated we should expect to see a relative increase in the hematocrit

Clinical implications

HIGH

Clinical Implication	Additional information
Asthma and emphysema	An increased HCT (>44 or 0.44 in women and >48 or 0.48 in men) is by no means a definitive diagnostic marker for asthma or emphysema. Due to the lack of optimum oxygenation of the blood, the body will increase the red blood cell count to increase the number of cells that can be oxygenated. The hematocrit will go up accordingly.
Polycythemia (relative or primary)	**Relative**: a polycythemia that is relative to the degree of hemo-concentration, i.e. **dehydration** **Primary**: Polycythemia vera- a myeloproliferative disease marked by an increase in all blood cells. The hematocrit will go up according to the increase in cell volume
Dehydration	If the hematocrit is increased suspect dehydration. Dehydration is a very common problem and should be factored into your blood chemistry and CBC analysis. **Please see special topic on page 90 for more details.** **Pattern:** Suspect a short-term (acute) dehydration if there is an increased HGB (>14.5 or 145 in women or 15 or 150 in men) and/or HCT (>44 or 0.44 in women and >48 or 0.48 in men) along with an increased RBC count (>4.5 in women and 4.9 in men). A relative increase in Sodium (>142) and Potassium (>4.5) can be noted as well. Suspect a long-term (chronic) dehydration if any of the above findings are accompanied by an increased Albumin (>5.0 or 50 g/L), increased BUN (>16 or 5.71 mmol/L), and/or serum Protein (> 7.4 or 74 g/L).
Spleen hyperfunction	May be seen when the hematocrit is above the optimum range.
Other conditions associated with increased hematocrit levels include	Vitamin B-6 anemia Diarrhea Adrenal dysfunction.

LOW

Clinical Implication	Additional information
Anemia	A condition in which there is a decreased amount of hemoglobin, a decreased number of circulating RBCs, and a decrease in the hematocrit. Anemia is a symptom not a disease, and the cause of an anemia must be sought out: • Deficiencies of iron and certain vitamins (B12, folate, B6, copper) • Blood loss • Increased destruction The following are some of the different nutritional types of anemia.
Anemia- Iron deficiency	This is the most prevalent anemia worldwide. The major causes are: 1. Dietary inadequacies 2. Malabsorption 3. Increased iron loss 4. Increased iron requirements, e.g. pregnancy **Patterns:** If there is a decreased HCT (<37 or 0.37 in women and 40 or 0.4 in men) and/or HGB (<13.5 or 135 g/L in women and <14 or 140 in men), MCH (<28), MCV (<82) and MCHC (<32), and a decreased serum iron (< 50 or 8.96 μmol/dL), ferritin (33 in men and 10 in women), % transferrin saturation, and an increased RDW (>13), then iron anemia is **probable**. If TIBC is increased (>350 or 62.7 μmol/dL), internal/microscopic bleeding is **possible**, and should be ruled out with reticulocyte count (>1), urinalysis, and/or stool analysis. Iron deficiency anemia may be secondary to hypochlorhydria if serum phosphorous is decreased (<3.0) and serum globulin is increased (>2.8) or decreased (<2.4). Some of the subjective indicators for iron need are: 1. Prolonged fatigue, particularly in pregnancy

	2. Blue sclera of the eyes
	3. Pica and a desire to chew ice
	4. Inability to tolerate cold
Anemia- B6 deficiency	B6 anemia is not very common but possible given the deficiencies of B6 and other B complex vitamins. **Pattern:** If there is a decreased HCT (<37 or 0.37 in women and 40 or 0.4 in men), HGB (<13.5 or 135 g/L in women and <14 or 140 in men), MCV (<82), MCH (<28), MCHC (<32), and an increased to normal serum iron (>100 or 17.91 μmol/dL) and/or ferritin (>236 in men and 122 in women), B6 anemia is **probable**. Look for a decreased SGOT/AST and/or SGPT/ALT and/or GGTP (<10)

> ## To receive master copies of our tracking forms and conversion tables please visit:
> # www.BloodChemistryAnalysis.com

| **B12/folic acid anemia** | **Pattern:**

 If there is a decreased HCT (<37 or 0.37 in women and 40 or 0.4 in men) with a decreased HGB (<13.5 or 135 g/L in women and <14 or 140 in men), RBC (<3.9 in women or 4.2 in men), and uric acid (<3.5 or 208 μmol/dL) and an increased MCH (>31.9), MCV (>90), RDW (>13), LDH (>200) (especially the LDH-1 isoenzyme fraction) and serum iron, then B12/folic acid anemia is **probable**.

 Often you will see decreased WBC (<5.0) and neutrophils (<40) and an increased LDH (>200) in megaloblastic anemia (i.e. anemia of large cells). Check with methylmalonic acid and homocysteine.

 The presence of hypersegmented neutrophils (5 or more lobes in more than 5% of all neutrophils) has been reported to be more sensitive and reliable than an elevated MCV in detecting megaloblastic anemia and is not affected by coexisting iron deficiency.

 If MCV is >97 oral supplementation may be ineffective. B12 injections may be needed. |

Copper anemia	**Pattern:** If there is decreased HCT (<37 or 0.37 in women and 40 or 0.4 in men) with a decreased HGB (<13.5 or 135 g/L in women and <14 or 140 in men) and RBCs (<3.9 in women or 4.2 in men), and low high MCV (>89.9), an increased to normal MCH (>31.9), and an increased or decreased hair copper, then copper anemia is **possible**. Check serum or WBC copper.
Internal bleeding	An unrecognized internal bleed can cause a gradual decrease in hematocrit due to the loss of blood. Internal bleeding is a serious condition and should be referred to a specialist qualified to diagnose and treat this condition.
Digestive inflammation	A decreased HCT (<37 or 0.37 in women and 40 or 0.4 in men) is by no means diagnostic for digestive inflammation (Crohn's disease, ileitis, colitis, gastritis, etc.) but one of a number of patterns seen with these disorders. **Pattern:** Decreased total globulin (<2.4 or 24 g/L), decreased serum phosphorous (<3.0 or 0.97 mmol/L), increased BUN (>16 or 5.71 mmol/L), while serum gastrin generally will be increased, basophils and ESR increased.
Thymus hypofunction	A hematocrit below the optimum range (<37 or 0.37 in women and 40 or 0.4 in men) is associated with thymus dysfunction. Indications of thymus hypofunction include: 1. Delayed healing time 2. Immune insufficiency 3. Frequent colds and flu 4. Chemical sensitivity
Vitamin C need	A decreased hematocrit level is associated with vitamin C need. **Pattern:** Albumin will frequently be decreased (<4.0 or 40g/L) along a decreased HCT (<37 or 0.37 in women and 40 or 0.4 in men), HGB (<13.5 or 135 g/L in women and <14 or 140 in men), MCH (<28), MCHC (<32), serum iron (< 50 or 8.96 µmol/dL). There will also be an increased MCV (>90), alkaline phosphatase (>100), fibrinogen, and RBCs (>4.5 in women and >4.9 in men).

	Both the lingual ascorbic acid test and Urinary vitamin C will generally be out of range. **Please see the special topic on the lingual ascorbic acid test below for more details.**

Lingual Ascorbic Acid Test

This test is an accurate, painless, and rapid method to determine the tissue levels of ascorbic acid in the body. The test uses an oxidation-reduction reaction between the ascorbic acid present in lingual tissues and 2,6 dichlorphenol-indophenol, a dye that will be rendered colorless when reduced by ascorbic acid. During this reaction ascorbic acid is converted into hydro-L-ascorbic acid.

This test has been shown to correlate with plasma levels, and is an accurate indicator for tissue levels of vitamin C and antioxidants.

Other conditions associated with decreased hematocrit levels include	Chronic intestinal parasites Free radical pathology Adrenal hypofunction	Thiamine deficiency Hereditary anemia Liver and renal dysfunction

Interfering Factors:

Falsely increased levels	Falsely decreased levels
• People living at high altitude will have an increased hematocrit • Dehydration • Infants: the normal value is higher for infants due to the large number of large (macrocytic) cells	• In iron deficiency anemia the red cells are smaller and therefore pack to a smaller volume causing a decreased HCT but often a normal RBC count • Females usually have a slightly lower hematocrit than males • Hematocrit will often be lower after age 60

Related Tests:

HGB, RBC, MCV, MCH, serum iron, serum ferritin, CBC or transferrin, total serum globulin (HCl need), reticulocyte count, alpha I and alpha 2 globulin (asthma and emphysema), total protein, and albumin (dehydration).

Hemoglobin

Discussion

Hemoglobin is the oxygen carrying molecule in red blood cells. The oxygen-combining capacity of the blood is directly proportional to the hemoglobin concentration. HGB is useful to determine the cause and type of anemia when viewed with other red blood cell indices and iron values (HCT, RBC, MCV, MCH, serum ferritin, serum iron and TIBC)

Often patients with low normal serum iron, serum ferritin, HGB, and HCT are generally more active and healthy than those patients with high normal or increased values.

Ranges:

	Standard U.S. Units	**Standard International Units**
Conventional Laboratory Range	**Males**: 12.5 – 17.0 g/dl **Females**: 11.5 – 15.0 g/dl	**Males**: 125 – 170 g/L **Females**: 115 – 150 g/L
Optimal Range	**Males**: 14.0 – 15.0 g/dl **Females**: 13.5 – 14.5 g/dl	**Males**: 140 – 150 g/L **Females**: 135 – 145 g/L
Alarm Ranges	< 10.0 or > 17.0 g/dl	< 100 or > 170 g/L

When would you run this test?

1. Determining degree of anemia and polycythemia: Although it cannot tell you the type of anemia the hemoglobin, along with RBC count and hematocrit, can help determine the degree of anemia and polycythemia

2. Evaluating treatment of anemia: As an anemia is treated we should expect to see a relative increase in the hemoglobin

3. Screen for dehydration

Clinical implications

HIGH

Clinical Implication	Additional information
Asthma and emphysema	An increased hemoglobin (>14.5 or 145 in women or 15 or 150 in men) is by no means a definitive diagnostic marker for asthma or emphysema. Due to the lack of optimum oxygenation of the blood, the body will increase the red blood cell count to increase the number of cells that can be oxygenated. The hemoglobin will go up accordingly.
Polycythemia **(relative or primary)**	**Relative**: a polycythemia that is relative to the degree of hemoconcentration, i.e. **dehydration.** **Primary**: Polycythemia vera- a myeloproliferative disease marked by an increase in all blood cells. The hemoglobin will go up according to the increase in cell volume.
Dehydration	If the hemoglobin is increased suspect dehydration. Dehydration is a very common problem and should be factored into your blood chemistry and CBC analysis. **Please see special topic on page 90 for more details.** **Pattern:** ⬦ Suspect a short-term (acute) dehydration if there is an increased HGB (>14.5 or 145 in women or 15 or 150 in men) and/or HCT (>44 or 0.44 in women and >48 or 0.48 in men) along with an increased RBC count (>4.5 in women and >4.9 in men). A relative increase in Sodium (>142) and Potassium (>4.5) can be noted as well. ⬦ Suspect a long-term (chronic) dehydration if any of the above findings are accompanied by an increased Albumin (>5.0 or 50 g/L), increased BUN (>16 or 5.71 mmol/L), and/or serum Protein (> 7.4 or 74 g/L).
Drug causes of ⬆	✳ Gentamicin ✳ Methyldopa
Other conditions associated with increased hemoglobin levels include	⬦ Vitamin B-6 anemia ⬦ Diarrhea ⬦ Adrenal dysfunction.

LOW

Clinical Implication	Additional information
Anemia	A condition in which there is a decreased amount of hemoglobin, a decreased number of circulating RBCs, and a decrease in the hematocrit. Anemia is a symptom not a disease, and the cause of an anemia must be sought out: • Deficiencies of iron and certain vitamins (B12, folate, B6) • Blood loss • Increased destruction The following are some of the different common types.
Anemia- Iron deficiency	This is the most prevalent anemia worldwide. The major causes are: 1. Dietary inadequacies 2. Malabsorption 3. Increased iron loss 4. Increased iron requirements **Patterns:** If there is a decreased HGB (<13.5 or 135 g/L in women and <14 or 140 in men) and/or HCT (<37 or 0.37 in women and 40 or 0.4 in men), MCH (<28), MCV (<82), and MCHC (32), and a decreased serum iron (< 50 or 8.96 µmol/dL), ferritin (<33 in men or 10 in women), % transferrin saturation, and an increased RDW (>13), then iron anemia is **probable**. If TIBC is increased (>350 or 62.7 µmol/dL), microscopic bleeding is **possible**, and should be ruled out with reticulocyte count, urinalysis, and/or stool analysis. Iron deficiency anemia may be secondary to hypochlorhydria if serum phosphorous is decreased (<3.0 or 0.97 mmol/L) and serum globulin is increased (>2.8 or 28 g/L) or decreased (<2.4 or 24 g/L). Some of the subjective indicators for iron need are: 1. Prolonged fatigue, particularly in pregnancy. 2. Blue sclera of the eyes. 3. Pica and a desire to chew ice.

Anemia- B6 deficiency	B6 anemia is not very common but possible given the deficiencies of B6 and other B complex vitamins.
	Pattern:
	If there is a decreased HCT (<37 or 0.37 in women and 40 or 0.4 in men), HGB (<13.5 or 135 g/L in women and <14 or 140 in men), MCV (82), MCH (<28), MCHC (<32), and an increased to normal serum iron (>100 or 17.91 µmol/dL) and/or ferritin (>236 in men or 122 in women), B6 anemia is **probable**. Look for a decreased SGOT/AST and/or SGPT/ALT and/or GGTP (<10).
Anemia- B12/folic acid deficiency	**Pattern:**
	If there is a decreased HGB (<13.5 or 135 g/L in women and <14 or 140 in men) with a decreased HCT (<37 or 0.37 in women and 40 or 0.4 in men), RBC (<3.9 in women or 4.2 in men), and uric acid (<3.5 or 208 µmol/dL) and an increased MCH (> 31.9), MCV (>89.9), RDW (>13), LDH (>200) (especially the LDH-1 isoenzyme fraction,) and serum iron, then B12/folic acid anemia is **probable**.
	Often you will see decreased WBC (<5.0) and neutrophils (<40) and an increased LDH (>200) in megaloblastic anemia (i.e. anemia of large cells). Check with methylmalonic acid and homocysteine.
	The presence of hypersegmented neutrophils (5 or more lobes in more than 5% of all neutrophils) has been reported to be more sensitive and reliable than an elevated MCV in detecting megaloblastic anemia and is not affected by coexisting iron deficiency. If MCV is >97 oral supplementation may be ineffective. B12 injections may be needed.
Copper anemia	If there is decreased HGB (<13.5 or 135 g/L in women and <14 or 140 in men) with a decreased HCT (<37 or 0.37 in women and 40 or 0.4 in men) and RBCs (<3.9 in women or 4.2 in men), and low high MCV (>89.9), an increased to normal MCH (>31.9), and an increased or decreased hair copper, then copper anemia is **possible**. Check serum or WBC copper.
Vitamin C need	A decreased hemoglobin level is associated with vitamin C need.
	Pattern:
	Albumin will frequently be decreased (<4.0 or 40g/L) along a decreased HCT (<37 or 0.37 in women and 40 or 0.4 in

	men), HGB (<13.5 or 135 g/L in women and <14 or 140 in men), MCH (<28), MCHC (<32), serum iron (< 50 or 8.96 μmol/dL). There will also be an increased MCV (>90), alkaline phosphatase (>100), fibrinogen, and RBCs (>4.5 in women and >4.9 in men).
	Both the lingual ascorbic acid test and Urinary vitamin C will generally be out of range. **Please see the special topic on the lingual ascorbic acid test on page 218 for more details.**
Digestive inflammation	A decreased HGB (<13.5 or 135 g/L in women and <14 or 140 in men) is by no means diagnostic for digestive inflammation (Crohn's disease, ileitis, colitis, gastritis, etc.) but one of a number of patterns seen with these disorders.
	<u>Pattern</u>:
	Decreased total globulin (<2.4 or 24 g/L), decreased serum phosphorous (<3.0 or 0.97 mmol/L), increased BUN (>16 or 5.71 mmol/L), while serum gastrin generally will be increased, basophils (>1) and ESR increased.
Internal bleeding	An unrecognized internal bleed can cause a gradual decrease in hemoglobin due to the loss of blood.
	Internal bleeding is a serious condition and should be referred to a specialist qualified to diagnose and treat this condition.
Other conditions associated with decreased hemoglobin levels include	Chronic intestinal parasites Free radical pathology Adrenal hypofunction Thiamine deficiency Hereditary anemia Liver and renal dysfunction

Interfering Factors:

Falsely increased levels	Falsely decreased levels
• People living at high altitudes will have increased values • Higher in infants	• Excessive fluid intake • Pregnancy • Drugs: there are many drugs that will cause a decreased hemoglobin

Related Tests:

HCT, RBC, MCV, MCH, serum iron, serum ferritin, RBC or transferrin, total serum globulin HCl need), reticulocyte count, alpha I and alpha 2 globulin (asthma and emphysema), total protein, and albumin (dehydration).

Mean Corpuscular Volume

Discussion

Mean Corpuscular Volume (MCV) is one of the red blood cell indices used to differentiate anemia. The MCV is a measurement of the volume in cubic microns of an average single red blood cell. MCV indicates whether the red blood cell size appears normal (normocytic), small (microcytic), or large (macrocytic).

- An increase or decrease in MCV can help determine the type of anemia present. It should always be considered along with the MCH when determining whether or not a patient has a vitamin B-6, vitamin B-12, or folic acid anemia.

- If the MCV is greater than 89.9 cubic microns, the red cells are macrocytic; if the MCV is less than 82.0 cubic microns, the red cells are microcytic; if the MCV is within the optimum range, the red cells are normocytic.

- MCV may be normal in concomitant folate and iron deficiency anemia

Ranges:

	Standard U.S. Units	Standard International Units
Conventional Laboratory Range	$80.0 - 98.0 \ \mu^3$	80.0 – 98.0 fL
Optimal Range	$82.0 - 89.9 \ \mu^3$	82.0 – 89.9 fL
Alarm Ranges	$<78.0 \ or \ >95.5 \ \mu^3$	<78.0 or >95.5 fL

When would you run this test?

1. Determining type of anemia: by assessing the size of the cell, along with other red cell indices, the true cause of a person's anemia can be determined.

Clinical implications

HIGH (Macrocytosis)

Clinical Implication	Additional information
Anemia- Vitamin B12 and/or folic acid deficiency	B12 and folic acid are needed for proper nucleus development. In situations of deficiency the cytoplasm of the erythrocyte continues to expand until the nucleus has reached its proper size. This leads to large red blood cells.Deficiency may occur for a number of different reasons: • **Decreased ingestion:** vegan diet. • **Impaired absorption:** Intrinsic factor deficiency, pernicious anemia, malabsorption, HCl need, hypochlorhydria. • **Competitive parasites:** fish tape worm infestations. • **Increased requirements:** Chronic pancreatic disease, pregnancy, hyperthyroidism. • **Impaired utilization:** enzyme deficiencies, abnormal binding proteins. **Pattern:** The probability of vitamin B-12 or folate deficiency anemia increases when the MCV is increased (>90) and the MCH is above 31.9. If there is also an increased RDW (>13), MCHC (>35), and LDH (>200) (especially the LDH-1 isoenzyme fraction), and a decreased uric acid level the probability of vitamin B-12 or folic acid anemia is very high. Serum or urinary methylmalonic acid is a good test for confirming vitamin B-12 deficiency. A serum or urinary homocysteine can help confirm folic acid and vitamin B-6 deficiency. The presence of hypersegmented neutrophils (5 or more lobes in more than 5% of all neutrophils) has been reported to be more sensitive and reliable than an elevated MCV in detecting megaloblastic anemia and is not affected by coexisting iron deficiency.
Hypochlorhydria	Hypochlorhydria is **possible** with an increased MCV, MCHC and/or MCH, especially with a low serum iron and an increased (>2.8 or 28 g/L) or decreased (<2.4 or 24 g/L) total globulin. Hypochlorhydria is **probable** if BUN is increased (>16 or 5.71

	mmol/L) and/or serum phosphorous is decreased (<3.0 or 0.97 mmol/L). **Please see the special topic on Hypochlorhydria on page 96 for more details.**
Vitamin C need	An increased MCV level is associated with vitamin C need. **Pattern:** 🍂 Albumin will frequently be decreased (<4.0 or 40g/L) along a decreased HCT (<37 or 0.37 in women and 40 or 0.4 in men), HGB (<13.5 or 135 g/L in women and <14 or 140 in men), MCH (<28), MCHC (<32), serum iron (< 50 or 8.96 μmol/dL). There will also be an increased MCV (>89.9), alkaline phosphatase (>100), fibrinogen and RBCs (>4.5 in women and >4.9 in men). Both the lingual ascorbic acid test and Urinary vitamin C will generally be out of range. **Please see the special topic on the lingual ascorbic acid test on page 218 for more details.**
Other conditions associated with increased MCV levels include	❇ Hereditary anemia

LOW (Microcytosis)

Clinical Implication	Additional information
Iron deficiency anemia	This is the most prevalent anemia worldwide. The major causes are: 1. Dietary inadequacies 2. Malabsorption 3. Increased iron loss 4. Increased iron requirements **Patterns:** ❇ If there is a decreased MCH (<28), MCV (<82), MCHC (<32), and HCT (<37 or 0.37 in women and 40 or 0.4 in men) and/or HGB (<13.5 or 135 g/L in women and <14 or 140 in men), and a decreased serum iron (< 50 or 8.96 μmol/dL), ferritin (<33 in men or 10 in women), % transferrin saturation, and ↑ RDW (>13), then iron anemia is **probable**.

	✴ If TIBC is increased (>350 or 62.7 µmol/dL), microscopic bleeding is **possible**, and should be ruled out with reticulocyte count, urinalysis, and/or stool analysis. 🌰 Iron deficiency anemia may be secondary to hypochlorhydria if serum phosphorous is decreased (<3.0 or 0.97 mmol/L) and serum globulin is increased (>2.8 or 28 g/L) or decreased (<2.4 or 24 g/L). Some of the subjective indicators for iron need are: 1. Prolonged fatigue, particularly in pregnancy 2. Blue sclera of the eyes 3. Pica and a desire to chew ice 4. Inability to tolerate cold
Anemia- B6 deficiency	B6 anemia is not very common but possible given the deficiencies of B6 and other B complex vitamins. **Pattern:** 🌰 If there is a decreased MCV (<82), MCH (<28), MCHC (<32), HGB (<13.5 or 135 g/L in women and <14 or 140 in men), and/or HCT (<37 or 0.37 in women and 40 or 0.4 in men) and an increased or normal serum iron (>100 or 17.91 µmol/dL) and/or ferritin (>236 in men and 122 in women), B6 anemia is **possible**. 🌰 If ↓there is a decreased MCV (<82), MCH (<28), and normal serum iron/ferritin, with a decreased SGOT/AST, SGPT/ALT or GGTP (<10), B6 anemia is **probable**.
Internal bleeding	An internal bleed can slowly deplete the body of iron due to the loss of red blood cells causing a decreased MCV. Internal bleeding is a serious condition and should be referred to a specialist qualified to diagnose and treat this condition.
Other conditions associated with decreased MCV levels include	🌰 Intestinal parasites 🌰 Heavy-metal body burdens	🌰 Free radical pathology 🌰 Iron anemia secondary to digestive inflammation or hypochlorhydria.

Interfering Factors:

Falsely increased levels	Falsely decreased levels
• May be increased with a high white blood cell count • May be increased with high reticulocyte count • Newborns • May be ↑ in autoagglutination	• None noted

Related Tests:

Serum or urinary methylmalonic acid and homocysteine, MCH, serum iron, serum ferritin, HGB, HCT, RBC, TIBC, or % transferrin saturation. The suspicion of vitamin B-6, vitamin B-12, or folic acid anemia should be confirmed with a serum or urinary methylmalonic acid and serum or urinary homocysteine.

Mean Corpuscular Hemoglobin

Discussion

 The Mean Corpuscular Hemoglobin (MCH) is a calculated value and is an expression of the average weight of hemoglobin per red blood cell. MCH, along with MCV can be helpful in determining the type of anemia present.

- An increase or decrease in MCH can help determine the type of anemia present. It should always be considered along with the MCV when determining whether or not a patient has a vitamin B-6, vitamin B-12, or folic acid anemia.

- Serum or urinary methylmalonic acid is a good test for confirming vitamin B-12 deficiency. A serum or urinary homocysteine can help confirm folic acid and vitamin B-6 deficiency.

Ranges:

	Standard U.S. Units	Standard International Units
Conventional Laboratory Range	27.0 – 34.0 pg	27.0 – 34.0 pg
Optimal Range	28.0 – 31.9 pg	28.0 – 31.9 pg
Alarm Ranges	<24.0 or > 34.0 pg	<24.0 or > 34.0 pg

When would you run this test?

1. To help determine cause of anemia: As one of the red blood cell indices the MCH is important in helping determine the cause of anemia, especially seriously anemic patients.

Clinical implications

HIGH

Clinical Implication	Additional information
Anemia- Vitamin B12 and/or folic acid deficiency	B12 and folic acid are needed for proper nucleus development. In situations of deficiency the cytoplasm of the erythrocyte continues to expand until the nucleus has reached its proper size. This leads to large red blood cells. Deficiency may occur for a number of different reasons: • **Decreased ingestion:** vegan diet. • **Impaired absorption:** Intrinsic factor deficiency, pernicious anemia, malabsorption, HCl need, hypochlorhydria. • **Competitive parasites:** fish tape worm infestations. • **Increased requirements:** Chronic pancreatic disease, pregnancy, hyperthyroidism. • **Impaired utilization:** enzyme deficiencies, abnormal binding proteins. **Pattern:** The probability of vitamin B-12 or folate deficiency anemia increases when the MCH is increased (>31.9) and there is an increased MCV (>90). If there is also an increased RDW (>13), MCHC (>34), and LDH (>200) (especially the LDH-1 isoenzyme fraction), and a decreased uric acid level (<3.5 or 208 μmol/dL) the probability of vitamin B-12 or folic acid anemia is very high. Serum or urinary methylmalonic acid is a good test for confirming vitamin B-12 deficiency. A serum or urinary homocysteine can help confirm folic acid and vitamin B-6 deficiency. The presence of hypersegmented neutrophils (5 or more lobes in more than 5% of all neutrophils) has been reported to be more sensitive and reliable than an elevated MCV in detecting megaloblastic anemia and is not affected by coexisting iron deficiency.
Hypochlorhydria	Hypochlorhydria is **possible** with an increased MCH (>31.9), MCV (>90), and/or MCHC (>34), especially with a low serum iron (< 50 or 8.96 μmol/dL) and an increased (>2.8 or 28 g/L) or decreased (<2.4 or 24 g/L) total globulin.

	Hypochlorhydria is **probable** if BUN is increased (>16 or 5.71 mmol/L) and/or serum phosphorous is decreased (<3.0 or 0.97 mmol/L). **Please see the special topic on Hypochlorhydria on page 96 for more details.**
Other conditions associated with increased MCH levels include	✳ Hereditary anemia

LOW

Clinical Implication	Additional information
Anemia- Iron deficiency	This is the most prevalent anemia worldwide. The major causes are: 1. Dietary inadequacies 2. Malabsorption 3. Increased iron loss 4. Increased iron requirements **Patterns:** ✳ If there is a decreased MCH (<28), MCV (<82), MCHC (<32), and HCT (<37 or 0.37 in women and 40 or 0.4 in men) and/or HGB (<13.5 or 135 g/L in women and <14 or 140 in men), and a decreased serum iron (< 50 or 8.96 μmol/dL), ferritin (<33 in men or 10 in women), % transferrin saturation, and ↑ RDW (>13), then iron anemia is **probable**. ✳ If TIBC is increased (>350 or 62.7 μmol/dL), microscopic bleeding is **possible**, and should be ruled out with reticulocyte count, urinalysis, and/or stool analysis. 🍂 Iron deficiency anemia may be secondary to hypochlorhydria if serum phosphorous is decreased (<3.0 or 0.97 mmol/L) and serum globulin is increased (>2.8 or 28 g/L) or decreased (<2.4 or 24 g/L). Some of the subjective indicators for iron need are: 1. Prolonged fatigue, particularly in pregnancy 2. Blue sclera of the eyes

	3. Pica and a desire to chew ice 4. Inability to tolerate cold
Anemia- B6 deficiency	B6 anemia is not very common but possible given the deficiencies of B6 and other B complex vitamins. **Pattern:** 🌰 If there is a decreased MCV (<82), MCH (<28), MCHC (<32), HGB (<13.5 or 135 g/L in women and <14 or 140 in men), and/or HCT (<37 or 0.37 in women and 40 or 0.4 in men) and an increased or normal serum iron (>100 or 17.91 μmol/dL) and/or ferritin (>236 in men and 122 in women), B6 anemia is **possible**. 🌰 If there is a decreased MCV (<82), MCH (<28) and normal serum iron/ferritin, with a decreased SGOT/AST, SGPT/ALT, or GGTP (<10), B6 anemia is **probable**.
Internal bleeding	An internal bleed can slowly deplete the body of iron due to the loss of red blood cells causing a decreased MCH. Internal bleeding is a serious condition and should be referred to a specialist qualified to diagnose and treat this condition.
Heavy metal body burden (e.g. lead, aluminum, cadmium and other toxic metals)	One of the significant effects of toxic metals is the impact they have on red blood cells especially hemoglobin. **Pattern:** 🌰 If there is a decreased MCH (<28) and MCHC (<32) with an increased Uric acid (>5.9 or > 351 μmol/dL), suspect a heavy metal body burden. Confirm with a hair analysis or toxic element testing via blood or urine. The serum levels of the metals may also be increased, but in sub-acute conditions the serum levels may be normal. A heavy metal body burden will appear in a hair analysis or urinary/whole blood element tests before an increase is seen in the serum.
Vitamin C need	A decreased MCH level (<28) is associated with vitamin C need. **Pattern:** 🌰 Albumin will frequently be decreased (<4.0 or 40g/L)along a decreased HCT (<37 or 0.37 in women and 40 or 0.4 in men), HGB (<13.5 or 135 g/L in women and <14 or 140 in men), MCH (<28), MCHC (<32), serum iron (< 50 or 8.96 μmol/dL). There will also be an increased MCV (>90),

	alkaline phosphatase (>100), fibrinogen, and RBCs (>4.5 in women and >4.9 in men).
	Both the lingual ascorbic acid test and Urinary vitamin C will generally be out of range. **Please see the special topic on the lingual ascorbic acid test on page 218 more details.**
Less common causes of MCH decrease	🩸 Intestinal parasites 🩸 Free radical pathology ✹ Rheumatoid arthritis

Interfering Factors:

Falsely increased levels	Falsely decreased levels
• Hyperlipidemia • WBC counts > 50,000 will falsely raise the hemoglobin value, and this will falsely raise the MCH • High heparin values	• None noted

Related Tests:

Serum or urinary methylmalonic acid and homocysteine, MCV, serum iron, serum ferritin, HGB, HCT, RBC, TIBC or transferrin.

Mean Corpuscular Hemoglobin Concentration
MCHC

Discussion

The Mean Corpuscular Hemoglobin Concentration (MCHC) measures the average concentration of hemoglobin in the red blood cells. It is a calculated value.

- **NOTE:** It is important to remember that no MCHC occurs over 37 g/dl because RBCs cannot accommodate more than 37 g/dl of hemoglobin

Ranges:

	Standard U.S. Units	Standard International Units
Conventional Laboratory Range	32.0 – 36.0 g/dl	0.32 – 0.36
Optimal Range	32.0 – 35.0 g/dl	0.32 – 0.35

When would you run this test?

1. Monitoring anemia therapy: The MCHC is most valuable in monitoring therapy for anemia because it uses the 2 most accurate hematological determinations (HCT and HGB) in its calculation.

Clinical implications

HIGH

Clinical Implication	Additional information
Anemia- Vitamin B12 and/or folic acid deficiency	B12 and folic acid are needed for proper nucleus development. In situations of deficiency the cytoplasm of the erythrocyte continues to expand until the nucleus has reached its proper size. This leads to large red blood cells. Deficiency may occur for a number of different reasons: • **Decreased ingestion:** vegan diet.

	• **Impaired absorption:** Intrinsic factor deficiency, pernicious anemia, malabsorption, HCl need, hypochlorhydria.
	• **Competitive parasites:** fish tape worm infestations.
	• **Increased requirements:** Chronic pancreatic disease, pregnancy, hyperthyroidism.
	• **Impaired utilization:** enzyme deficiencies, abnormal binding proteins.
	Pattern:
	If the MCHC is increased (>34) and there is an increased MCH (>31.9) in conjunction with an increased MCV (> 90), an increased RDW (>13), LDH (>200) (especially the LDH-1 isoenzyme fraction), and a decreased uric acid level (<3.5 or 208 µmol/dL), the probability of vitamin B-12 or folic acid anemia is very high.
	This finding should be confirmed with a serum or urinary methylmalonic acid (vitamin B-12) and serum or urinary homocysteine (folic acid and vitamin B-6).
	The presence of hypersegmented neutrophils (5 or more lobes in more than 5% of all neutrophils) has been reported to be more sensitive and reliable than an elevated MCV in detecting megaloblastic anemia and is not affected by coexisting iron deficiency.
Hypochlorhydria	Hypochlorhydria is **possible** with an increased MCHC (>34), MCH (>31.2), and/or MCV (>90), especially with a low serum iron (< 50 or 8.96 µmol/dL) and an increased (>2.8 or 28 g/L) or decreased (<2.4 or 24 g/L) total globulin.
	Hypochlorhydria is **probable** if BUN is increased (>16 or 5.71 mmol/L) and/or serum phosphorous is decreased (<3.0 or 0.97 mmol/L).
	Please see the special topic on Hypochlorhydria on page 96 for more details.
Other conditions associated with increased MCHC levels include	❀ Hereditary anemia

LOW

Clinical Implication	Additional information
Vitamin C need	A decreased MCHC level (<32)is associated with vitamin C need. **Pattern:** Albumin will frequently be decreased (<4.0 or 40g/L) along a decreased HCT (<37 or 0.37 in women and 40 or 0.4 in men), HGB (<13.5 or 135 g/L in women and <14 or 140 in men), MCH (<28), serum iron (< 50 or 8.96 µmol/dL). There will also be an increased MCV (>90), alkaline phosphatase (>100), fibrinogen. Both the lingual ascorbic acid test and Urinary vitamin C will generally be out of range. **Please see the special topic on the lingual ascorbic acid test on page 218 for more details.**
Anemia- B6 deficiency	B6 anemia is not very common but possible given the deficiencies of B6 and other B complex vitamins. **Pattern:** If there is a decreased MCV (<82), MCH (<28), MCHC (<32), HGB (<13.5 or 135 g/L in women and <14 or 140 in men), and/or HCT (<37 or 0.37 in women and 40 or 0.4 in men) and an increased or normal serum iron (>100 or 17.91 µmol/dL) and/or ferritin (>236 in men and 122 in women), B6 anemia is **possible**. If there is a decreased MCV (<82), MCH (<28), and normal serum iron/ferritin, with a decreased SGOT/AST, SGPT/ALT or GGTP (<10), B6 anemia is **probable**.
Anemia- Iron deficiency	This is the most prevalent anemia worldwide. The major causes are: 1. Dietary inadequacies 2. Malabsorption 3. Increased iron loss 4. Increased iron requirements **Patterns:** If there is a decreased MCH (<28), MCV (<82), MCHC (<32), and HCT (<37 or 0.37 in women and 40 or 0.4 in

	men) and/or HGB (<13.5 or 135 g/L in women and <14 or 140 in men), and a decreased serum iron (< 50 or 8.96 μmol/dL), ferritin (<33 in men or 10 in women), % transferrin saturation, and ↑ RDW (>13), then iron anemia is **probable**.
	If TIBC is increased (>350 or 62.7 μmol/dL), microscopic bleeding is **possible**, and should be ruled out with reticulocyte count, urinalysis, and/or stool analysis.
	Iron deficiency anemia may be secondary to hypochlorhydria if serum phosphorous is decreased (<3.0 or 0.97 mmol/L) and serum globulin is increased (>2.8 or 28 g/L) or decreased (<2.4 or 24 g/L).
	Some of the subjective indicators for iron need are:
	1. Prolonged fatigue, particularly in pregnancy
	2. Blue sclera of the eyes
	3. Pica and a desire to chew ice
	4. Inability to tolerate cold
Heavy metal body burden (e.g. lead, aluminum, cadmium, and other toxic metals)	One of the significant effects of toxic metals is the impact they have on red blood cells, especially hemoglobin.
	Pattern:
	If there is a decreased MCH (<28) and MCHC (<32) with a decreased uric acid (<3.5 or 208 μmol/dL), suspect a heavy metal body burden.
	Confirm with a hair analysis or toxic element testing via blood or urine. The serum levels of the metals may also be increased, but in sub-acute conditions the serum levels may be normal. The hair and urinary/blood tests will frequently reflect the increase before it is seen outside the reference range in the serum.
Other conditions associated with decreased MCHC levels include	Internal bleeding
	Thalassemia

Interfering Factors:

Falsely increased levels	Falsely decreased levels
• Hyperlipidemia	• None Noted
• Rouleaux formation in the blood	
• High heparin concentrations	

Related Tests:

Serum or urinary methylmalonic acid and homocysteine, MCH, serum iron, serum ferritin, HGB, HCT, RBC, TIBC, or transferrin.

The suspicion of vitamin B-6, vitamin B-12, or folic acid anemia should be confirmed with a serum or urinary methylmalonic acid and serum or urinary homocysteine.

Red Cell Distribution Width

Discussion

The Red Cell Distribution Width (RDW) is essentially an indication of the degree of anisocytosis (abnormal variation in size of red blood cells). It is not a helpful test for those who do not have anemia. It is helpful in the investigation of hematological disorders and monitoring therapy. Although the RDW will increase with vitamin BI2 deficiency, folic acid, and iron anemia, it is increased most frequently with vitamin B12 deficiency anemia.

Ranges:

	Standard U.S. Units	Standard International Units
Conventional Laboratory Range	11.7 – 15.0%	11.7 – 15.0%
Optimal Range	<13.0%	<13.0%

When would you run this test?

1. To investigate hematological disorders and monitor therapy

2. To help distinguish uncomplicated heterozygous thalassemia (Decreased MCV, normal RDW) from iron deficiency (decreased MCV, increased RDW)

3. Helpful in distinguishing anemia of chronic disease (normal RDW) from early iron deficiency anemia (low normal MCV, increased RDW)

NOTE: It is not a helpful test for those who do not have anemia

Clinical implications

HIGH

Clinical Implication	Additional information
Some conditions associated with increased RDW levels	Iron deficiency B12/folate deficiency

include	❈ Pernicious anemia (RDW of 12.9%)
	❈ Thalassemia
	Please check MCH, CMV, MCHC, HGB, HCT, RBC, Serum iron, and serum ferritin to determine the type of anemia

LOW

Clinical Implication	Additional information
Some conditions associated with decreased RDW levels include	❈ Post-hemorrhagic anemia (RDW of 9.9%)

Interfering Factors:

Falsely increased levels	Falsely decreased levels
• None Noted	• None Noted

Related Tests:

MCV, MCH, HGB, HCT, RBC, serum iron, serum ferritin, serum or urinary methylmalonic acid or homocysteine, TIBC, or % transferrin saturation.

Neutrophils

Discussion

Neutrophils are the white blood cells used by the body to combat bacterial or pyrogenic infections. They are the most numerous and important white cell in the body's reaction to inflammation. They are a primary defense against microbial infections via the process of phagocytosis.

- They have granules of enzymes and pyrogenes in their cytoplasm and in some cases can cause tissue damage with their release.

- In their immature stage of development, neutrophils are referred to as "bands". Please see the section on "bands" for a more in depth discussion.

Ranges: The following ranges are expressed as a % of the total WBC count

	Standard U.S. Units	**Standard International Units**
Conventional Laboratory Range	35 – 74%	35 – 74%
Optimal Range	40 – 60%	40 – 60%
Alarm Ranges	<30% or >80%	<30% or >80%

When would you run this test?
1. To more specifically screen the body's defense system
2. To detect the reason for an increased or decreased total WBC count: infections (bacterial and viral) and inflammation.

Clinical implications

HIGH (Neutrophilia)

Clinical Implication	Additional information
Childhood diseases (Measles, Mumps, Chicken-pox, Rubella, etc.)	The pattern seen in the Neutrophil count is as follows: **Neutrophils**: increased early (>60), decreased later (<40)
Acute, localized, and general bacterial infections	Neutrophils will be increased (>60). They are the primary cell type for fighting bacterial infections.

Acute viral infection	Neutrophils will tend to be normal	
Chronic viral or bacterial infection	Frequently an increased neutrophil count (>60) is seen with a decreased total WBC count (<5.0) in chronic infection.	
Inflammation	An increased neutrophil count (>60) will often be seen in acute and chronic inflammation (RA, SLE, Rheumatic fever and acute gout)	
Other conditions associated with increased neutrophil levels include	Intestinal parasites Free radical pathology (neoplasm) Adrenal dysfunction Late pregnancy	Asthma Emphysema Polycythemia Influenza with secondary bacterial infection

LOW (Neutropenia)

Clinical Implication	Additional information	
Blood diseases	Anything that affects the output of white blood cells from the bone marrow can cause a decreased neutrophil count (aplastic anemia, pernicious anemia, acute lymphoblastic leukemia)	
Chronic viral infection	A chronic viral infection is **possible** with decreased Neutrophils (<40) and increased Lymphocytes (>44), and or decreased total WBC count (<5.0).	
Other conditions associated with decreased neutrophil levels include	Hepatitis Free radical diseases (neoplasm) Vitamin B-12, vitamin B-6, and folic acid anemia Anterior pituitary dysfunction	Adrenal dysfunction Parathyroid hyperfunction Intestinal parasites (chronic) Rheumatoid arthritis Multiple food allergies

Interfering Factors:

Falsely increased levels	Falsely decreased levels
• Stress, excitement, and exercise can cause a temporary neutrophilia • Steroid administration: neutrophilia peaks in 4-6 hours • Children respond to infection with a greater rise in neutrophils than adults • Exposure to extreme cold or heat	• Exposure to extreme cold or heat • Elderly or weak people respond weakly or not at all to an infection • Myelosuppressive chemotherapy

Related Tests:
Total WBC count, differential count of WBCs, sedimentation rate

Bands

Discussion

Bands are young non-segmented neutrophils or metamylocytes. Bands are not usually seen in large numbers in the peripheral blood. They will be increased in acute infection even if there is no increase in the total WBC count. This increase in bands is known as a "shift to the left."

Ranges: The following ranges are expressed as a % of the total WBC count

	Standard U.S. Units	**Standard International Units**
Conventional Laboratory Range	0 – 10%	0 – 10%
Optimal Range	<5%	<5%
Alarm Ranges	>10%	>10%

When would you run this test?

1. The presence of bands can help determine the timing or severity of an infection.

2. The presence of band cells in a bacterial infection can often be a good prognosis.

Clinical implications

HIGH

Clinical Implication	Additional information
Active bacterial Infections	The presence of bands is an indication of a "regenerative" shift to the left and is often a good prognosis. Band cells are an excellent way to differentiate an active from a chronic viral or bacterial infection: • Band cells will generally increase in the active phase of an infection

	• Bands tend to normalize in the chronic or recovery phase
	Look for the site of the infection if not immediately obvious e.g. sinuses, middle ear, urinary tract.

Related Tests:

Total WBC count and differential

Lymphocytes

Discussion

Lymphocytes migrate to areas of inflammation in both the early and late stages of the inflammatory process. They are the source of immunoglobulins and of the cellular immune response where they play a role in immunological reactions.

● Lymphocytes are manufactured in the bone marrow and they migrate to other tissues to mature. Lymphocytes are used by the body to destroy and get rid of the toxic by-products of protein metabolism. When increased, excessive systemic toxins are possible, when decreased, infection is possible.

Ranges: The following ranges are expressed as a % of the total WBC count

	Standard U.S. Units	Standard International Units
Conventional Laboratory Range	14 – 46%	14 – 46%
Optimal Range	24 – 44%	24 – 44%
Alarm Ranges	<20% or >55%	<20% or >55%

When would you run this test?

1. To more specifically screen the body's defense system

2. To detect the reason for an increased or decreased total WBC count: infections (bacterial and viral) and inflammation

3. Relative lymphocytosis is present in various diseases and is often present with neutropenia

Clinical implications

HIGH (Lymphocytosis)

Clinical Implication	Additional information
Childhood diseases (Measles, Mumps, Chicken-pox, Rubella)	Lymphocytes will be decreased (<24) in early phase and increased in later phase (>44).

Acute viral infection	Lymphocytes will be increased (>44) along with an increased total WBC count (>7.5) in viral diseases such as upper respiratory infections, cytomegalovirus, infectious hepatitis, and toxoplasmosis.
Chronic viral infection	Increased lymphocytes (>44) with a decreased total WBC count (<5.0).
Infectious mononucleosis	A disease caused by the Epstein-Barr virus. It is most common in adolescents and young adults. It is characterized by an increased lymphocyte count (>10.5) and the presence of atypical lymphocytes or Downey cells. LDH levels are usually elevated in about 95% of cases of infectious mononucleosis and Epstein Barr infection (EBV). You may expect the following changes: decreased WBCs in first week, increased WBCs by 2nd week of illness, increased Alk phos and AST/SGOT (about 5-14 days after onset of illness), increased GGTP (about 7-21 days after onset of illness)
Acute bacterial infections	Lymphocytes will tend to be normal.
Inflammation	An increased lymphocyte count (>7.5) will often be seen in acute and chronic inflammation, especially Crohn's disease and ulcerative colitis.
Systemic toxicity or Poor Detoxification	Increased lymphocytes (>7.5) are associated with an increased level of toxicity in the body. If increased consider that either the body is dealing with excessive systemic toxins or the body cannot handle the current toxicity load and may not be detoxifying efficiently. Rule out heavy metals, xenobiotics, parasites, etc.
Other conditions associated with increased lymphocyte levels include	❄ Intestinal parasites ❄ Neoplasm 🖐 Adrenal dysfunction (hypoadrenalism) 🖐 Hypothyroidism ❄ Late pregnancy ❄ Asthma, emphysema ❄ Polycythemia ❄ Influenza with secondary bacterial infection

LOW (lymphopenia)

Clinical Implication	Additional information
Chronic viral or bacterial infection	Frequently a decreased lymphocyte count is seen with chronic infection, the classic case being the viral infection of AIDS.

Active infection	An active infection of unknown cause (i.e. not sure if it is bacterial or viral) can use up a large number of lymphocytes. Expect to see an increased total WBC count (> 7.5) and increased neutrophils (>60). Further testing should be considered (ESR, C reactive protein, etc.)	
Oxidative Stress and Free Radical Activity	Suspect excess free radical activity and oxidative stress if the lymphocyte count is decreased (<20). **Pattern:** If a decreased lymphocyte count (<20) is seen with a total cholesterol level suddenly below its historical level, a decreased albumin (<4.0 or 40 g/L) and low platelet levels (<150), an increased total globulin (>2.8 or 28 g/L) and uric acid level (>5.9 or > 351 μmol/dL), free radical pathology, which increases the risk for developing a neoplasm, should be investigated. This can be accomplished in the office using the Oxidata free radical test. **Please see page 152 for a discussion of this test.** Oxidative stress can cause an increased destruction of red blood cells; in these situations you will see an elevated bilirubin level. **Other tests include**: Acid Phosphatase, serum protein Electrophoresis, CEA, Anti-malignin Antibody, HCG, Alpha Fetoprotein, etc. If Alpha 1, Alpha 2, or gamma globulins are increased on a serum protein electrophoresis, free radical pathology should be investigated immediately.	
Suppressed bone marrow production	Anything that affects the output of white blood cells from the bone marrow can cause a decreased lymphocyte count (aplastic anemia, chemotherapy, radiation, Hodgkin's disease)	
Other conditions associated with decreased lymphocyte levels	Hepatitis Free radical diseases (neoplasm) Vitamin B-12, vitamin B-6 and folic acid anemia Anterior pituitary dysfunction	Adrenal dysfunction Parathyroid hyperfunction Intestinal parasites (chronic) Rheumatoid arthritis Multiple food allergies

Related Tests:

Total WBC count, differential count of WBCs, sedimentation rate, T and B lymphocyte Subset assay, immunoglobulins

Monocytes

Discussion

Monocytes are the body's second line of defense against infection. They are phagocytic cells that are capable of movement and remove dead cells, microorganisms, and particulate matter from circulating blood.

- Neutrophils are more active during the first 3 days of an inflammatory process. After that time they begin to break apart and the monocyte level will increase to phagocytize fragments of cells. Monocytes also produce the antiviral agent interferon.

Ranges: The following ranges are expressed as a % of the total WBC count

	Standard U.S. Units	Standard International Units
Conventional Laboratory Range	4 – 13%	4 – 13%
Optimal Range	<7%	<7%
Alarm Ranges	>15%	>15%

When would you run this test?

1. To follow the course of an infection
2. Monocytes are often elevated during the recovery phase of an infection

Clinical implications

HIGH

Clinical Implication	Additional information
Recovery phase of acute infection	Due to their phagocytic function monocytes are often the white blood cell that removes the bacterial, viral, and cellular residue of infection. It is a positive sign to see an increase in Monocytes (>7) towards the end of an infection.

Liver dysfunction	Not a primary marker but if an increased monocyte count (>7) is seen it is a good idea to rule out liver dysfunction. Functionally oriented liver problems, such as detoxification issues, liver congestion and conjugation problems are extremely common and should be evaluated based upon early prognostic indicators. The liver should always be viewed in the context of the hepato-biliary tree. Some of the key clinical indicators include: 1. Pain between shoulder blades 2. Stomach upset by greasy foods 3. If drinking alcohol, easily intoxicated 4. Headache over the eye 5. Sensitive to chemicals (perfume, cleaning solvents, insecticides, exhaust, etc.) 6. Hemorrhoids or varicose veins Check serum SGOT/AST, SGPT/ALT, GGTP, LDH, ALP, and bilirubin levels, especially if a chronic viral infection is suspected.
Intestinal parasites	If the monocyte count is elevated (>7) with increased eosinophils (>3) and increased basophils (>1), then intestinal parasites are **possible**. Further investigation is warranted, i.e. a digestive stool analysis with ova and parasite, especially if the subjective indicators are present. In some cases the stool tests may be normal especially with amoebic parasites or if the lab sample was not collected or analyzed appropriately by a qualified lab. Multiple and/or purged samples are sometimes necessary. **Please see the special topic on intestinal parasites on page 254 for more details.**
<u>**MALES**</u> **Urinary Tract Congestion:** • **Benign Prostatic Hypeertrophy (BPH)** 	An increased monocyte count (>7) may be associated with prostatic hypertrophy, especially If the serum creatinine is elevated (>1.1 or 97.2 µmol/dL) in a male over 40 years old. Often the creatinine will increase long before the PSA increases. <u>**Pattern:**</u> ☞ Suspect BPH if there is an increased creatinine level (>1.1 or 97.2 µmol/dL, along with a normal BUN and electrolytes.

	The likelihood of BPH increases when there is an increased creatinine level (>1.1 or 97.2 μmol/dL, along with a normal BUN and electrolytes, and an increased monocyte count (>7) and LDH isoenzyme #4, which has a prostatic origin.
	If BPH is suspected the following may be indicated: a microscopic examination of the urine for prostate cells, a urinalysis indicating infection, and a manual examination of the prostate
	Some of the key clinical indications of a developing prostate problem include:
	1. Difficulty urinating and/or dribbling
	2. Difficulty starting and stopping urine stream
	3. Waking to urinate at night
	4. Interruption of stream during urination
	5. Unresolved back pain and/or pain on inside of heels
	6. Feeling of incomplete bowel evacuation
	7. Erectile dysfunction

LOW

- Corticosteroid therapy will depress monocytes

- Not usually associated with any specific disease or disorder

Related Tests:

Total WBC count, WBC differential count

Basophils

Discussion

Basophils constitute a small percentage of the total white blood cell count. They are phagocytic and contain histamine, heparin, and serotonin in their cytoplasmic granules.

- They exist both in the blood and in the tissue where they are called mast cells. Similar to the basophils found in the blood, they store and produce histamine, serotonin, and heparin. Normally, mast cells are not found in peripheral blood.

- Basophils play an important role in the inflammatory process by releasing heparin and other substances to prevent clotting in the inflamed tissue. Basophils will often be increased with tissue inflammation.

Ranges: The following ranges are expressed as a % of the total WBC count

	Standard U.S. Units	**Standard International Units**
Conventional Laboratory Range	0 – 3%	0 – 3%
Optimal Range	0 – 1%	0 – 1%
Alarm Ranges	>5%	>5%

When would you run this test?

1. The basophil count is used to study allergic and inflammatory reactions.

2. There is a positive correlation between a high basophil count and a high concentration of histamine in the blood, though no cause and effect can be applied.

Clinical implications

HIGH

Clinical Implication	Additional information
Inflammation- non-specific	Any non-specific type of histamine, heparin, or serotonin-mediated inflammation or tissue destruction may be associated with an increased basophil count (>1) such as: bursitis, tendinitis, fibromyalgia, phlebitis, etc. With inflammation, basophils deliver heparin to the affected tissue to prevent clotting. With severe inflammation and subsequent tissue damage expect to see an increase in Alpha 1 globulin. If the inflammation is located in the digestive tract, bone, or liver expect to see increased Alkaline phosphatase levels (>100).
Intestinal parasites	Although not as indicative as an increased eosinophil count (>3), an increased basophil count (>1) is often seen with intestinal parasites, especially if inflammation is ruled-out as a cause of a basophil increase. Eosinophils may be normal with an intestinal amoebic problem; however, the basophil count may be increased. **Pattern:** If increased basophils (>1), increased eosinophils (>3), and increased monocytes (>7) intestinal parasites are **probable** and need to be ruled out with stool analysis. **Please see the special topic on intestinal parasites on page 254 for more information.**
Other conditions associated with increased basophil levels include	❋ Polycythemia ❋ Endocrine problems ❋ Influenza ❋ Chronic hemolytic anemia ⦿ Thyroid hypofunction

Related Tests:

C-Reactive Protein, erythrocyte sedimentation rate, serum protein electrophoresis (SPE), WBC and differential, total protein, RBC, and indices.

Eosinophils

Discussion

Eosinophils will be are often increased in patients that are suffering from intestinal parasites or food or environmental sensitivities/allergies. Eosinophils help remove and breakdown the by-products of protein catabolism. They have the ability to ingest antibody-antigen complexes and become active in later stages of inflammation. They are not effective against bacteria but do respond to allergic and parasitic disorders.

Ranges: The following ranges are expressed as a % of the total WBC count

	Standard U.S. Units	Standard International Units
Conventional Laboratory Range	0 – 7%	0 – 7%
Optimal Range	<3%	<3%

When would you run this test?

1. This test is used to screen for allergies, parasitic infections and to monitor treatment.

Clinical implications

HIGH

Clinical Implication	Additional information
Intestinal parasites	It is important to do further studies if the eosinophil count is increased (>3), i.e. a digestive stool analysis with ova and parasite, especially if the subjective indicators are present. In some cases the stool tests may be normal, especially with amoebic parasites or if the lab sample was not collected or analyzed appropriately by a qualified lab. Multiple and/or purged samples are sometimes necessary
	Pattern:
	If increased eosinophils (>3), increased basophils (>1), and increased monocytes (>7) intestinal parasites are **probable** and should be ruled out.
	Please see the special topic on intestinal parasites below for more information.

Intestinal Parasites

Intestinal parasites are a common problem, yet are difficult to diagnose. Those patients with the greater number of risk factors or poor digestive defenses should be considered for further stool analysis.

Risk factors

- The risk of parasite infection increases if your patients own house pets, or live/or work around farm animals.

- Parasites can be transmitted between family members.

- Foreign travel is a strong risk factor for intestinal parasites.

- Drinking untreated water, abroad or even in the U.S., where amoebas and Giardia are becoming more common.

- The risk increases with the consumption of raw meat or fish e.g. sushi, sashimi.

- Patients with poor digestion, especially hypochlorhydria, are at an increased risk for parasites due to the reduced digestive barriers to infection i.e. low stomach acid.

The following are some of the major subjective indicators of intestinal parasites. However, these are only a small number of the myriad of symptoms that can be present with undetected intestinal parasites.

- Chronic allergy/sensitivity.

- Dark circles under the eyes.

- **Digestive disorders**: chronic gas or bloating, chronic constipation or diarrhea, reduced or excessive appetite, burning or itching anus.

- **Dermatological disorders**: dry, scaly, itchy skin, dull or pallid complexion, prematurely aged skin.

- **Metabolic disorders**: difficulty gaining or losing weight, normal weight with large abdomen, chronic fatigue, wakes up groggy or fatigued.

- **Neurological**: chronic depression, Attention Deficit Disorder, hyper-activity (especially children).

Other: bites nails, picks nose, deep nocturnal cough (unproductive) very strong indication, dull eyes, nocturnal bruxism.

Food and Environmental allergy/sensitivity	An increased eosinophil count (>3) is associated with food allergies and/or sensitivities. There are a number of sophisticated and expensive tests for specific food allergies. These are often normal. In our experience a weekly diet diary can be a very helpful tool to investigate possible food allergies and sensitivities. An elimination diet for 4 weeks and a subsequent challenge of suspect foods can help determine the most common foods that a patient is allergic or sensitive to.
	Foods that the patient may be sensitive to most often are:
	• Dairy products
	• Gluten containing grains
	• Citrus
	• Shell fish
	• Foods containing additives and food dyes
	Patients should use the "Coca pulse testing" method or try an elimination challenge diet to successfully identify the main culprits. Several methods of food sensitivity testing are available.

Asthma	An increased eosinophil count (>3) is often seen in asthma due to the connection between allergies and asthma. A digestive stool analysis will frequently indicate dysbiosis in an asthmatic, and a liver detoxification panel will often indicate liver dysfunction.

Other conditions associated with increased Eosinophils levels include	❋ Neoplasm ❋ Adrenal dysfunction
	❋ Polycythemia ❋ Phlebitis
	❋ Thyroid hyperfunction ❋ Angio-neurotic edema
	❂ Anterior pituitary dysfunction ❋ Non-allergic rhinitis
	                                       ❋ Gastroenteritis
	                                       ❋ Eosinophilia myalgia syndrome

LOW

Stress	A decrease in the amount of circulating eosinophils is usually due to an increased adrenal steroid production that accompanies most conditions of bodily stress.

Interfering Factors:

Diurnal rhythm: Eosinophils follow a daily rhythm with the count being lowest in the morning, and rising from noon until midnight. Blood for serial eosinophil counts should be taken at the same time each day.

Falsely increased levels	Falsely decreased levels
• None noted	• Stressful situations such as burns, SLE, eclampsia, and postoperative states

Related Tests:

Digestive stool analysis to include ova and parasites, food allergy/sensitivity testing, food elimination plans, IgE, total WBC and differential, RBC and indices.

Blood Platelet count

Discussion

 Platelets or thrombocytes are the smallest of the formed elements in the blood. Platelets are necessary for blood clotting, vascular integrity, and vasoconstriction. They form adhesions and aggregates in the formation of a platelet plug, which plugs up breaks in small vessels.

● Platelet production is under the control of thrombopoietin. Platelets have a life-span between 8-10 days. Two-thirds of the platelets are found in circulating blood, the remaining one third is in the spleen.

● It is important to ask your patients about their use of drugs or supplements that are known to decrease platelet production before beginning therapy to increase their platelet count.

Ranges:

	Standard U.S. Units	Standard International Units
Conventional Laboratory Range	$155 - 385 \times 10^3/mm^3$	$155 - 385 \times 10^9/L$
Optimal Range	$155 - 385 \times 10^3/mm^3$	$155 - 385 \times 10^3/mm^3$
Alarm Ranges	<50 or $>700 \times 10^3/mm^3$	<50 or $>700 \times 10^9/L$

When would you run this test?

1. Evaluating bleeding disorders: Knowing the platelet count is helpful in the evaluation of bleeding disorders that occur in liver disease, thrombocytopenia and uremia

Clinical implications

HIGH

Clinical Implication	Additional information
Atherosclerosis	Platelet count may be high due to the platelet involvement in the plaque formation. People with atherosclerosis and

(leaf image)	atherosclerosis are often told they have "thick" blood and are advised by their medical doctors to take a baby aspirin to "thin" the blood.
	Pattern
	Atherosclerosis is **probable** if the platelet is increased (>350) along with an increased uric acid level (>5.9 or > 351 μmol/dL), an increased triglyceride (>200 or 2.26 mmol/L) in relation to total cholesterol (>220 or 5.69 mmol/L), a decreased HDL (<55 or 1.42 mmol/L) and an increased LDL (>120 or 3.1 mmol/L). C-reactive protein may also be elevated.
Purpura and petechiae	The platelet count may be high in these conditions.
Other conditions associated with increased platelet levels include	✦ Malignancies and chronic leukemias ✦ Polycythemia ✦ Inflammation: Inflammatory arthritis, acute infections ✦ Several types of anemia ✦ Oral contraceptives ✦ Acute blood loss ◉ Excessive antioxidant stress

LOW

Clinical Implication	Additional information
Infections	Some viral, rickettsial, and bacterial infections can cause a decreased platelet count (<150).
Idiopathic Thrombocytopenia (Rare image)	A hemorrhagic disease that is often triggered by a viral disease in children and has symptoms of purpura, ↑ platelet destruction, petechiae, mucosal bleeding, and thrombocytopenia. This is not something that you are likely to see in general practice.
Heavy metals (leaf image)	Blood platelets may be low (<150) when the body is dealing with an increased heavy metal load. Check for decreased MCH (<28), MCHC (<32), and LDH Isoenzyme #5. If either is decreased, along with a decreased platelet count (150), suspect a heavy metal body burden and consider hair analysis or toxic element testing via blood or urine.
Oxidative Stress and Free Radical Activity	Suspect excess free radical activity and oxidative stress if the platelet level is decreased. **Pattern:** ◉ If the platelet level is decreased (<150) along with a total

	cholesterol level that is suddenly below its historical and a decreased lymphocyte count (<20), a decreased albumin (<4.0 or 40 g/L) and an increased total globulin (>2.8 or 28 g/L) and uric acid level (>5.9 or > 351 μmol/dL), free radical pathology, which increases the risk for developing a neoplasm, should be investigated.
	This can be accomplished in the office using the Oxidata free radical test.
	Please see page 152 for a discussion of this test.
	Oxidative stress can cause an increased destruction of red blood cells; in these situations you will see an elevated bilirubin level.
	Other tests include: Acid Phosphatase, serum protein Electrophoresis, CEA, Anti-malignin Antibody, HCG, Alpha Fetoprotein, etc. If Alpha 1, Alpha 2, or gamma globulins are increased on a serum protein electrophoresis, free radical pathology should be investigated immediately.
Purpura and petechiae	The platelet count may be low in these conditions. People who bruise easily often have low vascular and capillary integrity. A low platelet count can exacerbate such a condition.
Drug causes of ↓	✼ Quinidine ✼ Heparin ✼ Gold salts ✼ Sulfas ✼ Digitoxin due to bone marrow suppression
Other conditions associated with decreased platelet levels include	✼ Neoplasm (especially leukemia) ✼ Liver dysfunction ✼ Several types of anemia (check RBC, HGB, HCT, MCV, MCH and serum iron or ferritin) 🌰 Sleep/wake cycle interruptions 　 🌰 Circadian rhythm dysfunction 🌰 Alcoholism 🌰 Deficiency of B12, folate, selenium, and/or iron 🌰 Excessive B3 supplementation

Interfering Factors:

Circadian rhythms: Platelet count is subject to circadian rhythms with the highest count occurring during the midday.

Children: Platelet counts> 500,000 are often present with healthy children.

Falsely increased levels	Falsely decreased levels
• High altitudes	• Normally decreased before menstruation
• After strenuous exercise	
• Excitement	
• In winter	

Related Tests:

WBC and differential, erythrocyte sedimentation rate, bleeding studies, platelet aggregation studies, C-Reactive Protein, total cholesterol, HDL. LDL and VLDL cholesterol, triglycerides, serum protein electrophoresis, RBC, HGB, HCT, MCV, and MCH.

APPENDIX

BLOOD CHEMISTRY AND COMPLETE BLOOD COUNT PATTERNS

Introduction

There are few diagnostic tests that are truly diagnostic all on their own. It is important to see the trends and patterns that exist between various tests. This section is organized to provide that information, and is broken into two sections.

Section One

The first section is a list of the individual components of the blood chemistry screen and complete blood count. Beside each component, organized by high or low values, is a list of the most common conditions seen with deviations from normal.

COMPONENT	HIGH/LOW	CONDITION
Glucose	High	• Insulin resistance • Early stage hyperglycemia/Diabetes • Metabolic Syndrome • Thiamine Need • Cortisol resistance • Fatty liver • Liver congestion
	Low	• Hypoglycemia- reactive • Hypoglycemia- Liver glycogen problem • Hyperinsulinism • Adrenal hypofunction
Hemoglobin A1C	High	• Diabetes mellitus • Insulin resistance
	Low	• Hypoglycemia
Triglycerides	High	• Metabolic Syndrome • Fatty liver • Liver congestion • Insulin resistance • Cardiovascular disease • Atherosclerosis • Poor metabolism and utilization of fats • Early stage hyperglycemia/Diabetes • Hyperlipidemia • Primary hypothyroidism • Adrenal cortical dysfunction • Secondary hypothyroidism- anterior pituitary dysfunction • Hyperlipoproteinemia • Alcoholism
	Low	• Liver/biliary dysfunction • Thyroid hyperfunction • Autoimmune processes • Adrenal hyperfunction

Blood Chemistry and CBC Interpretation- **Patterns**

COMPONENT	HIGH/LOW	CONDITION
Cholesterol	High	• Primary hypothyroidism • Adrenal cortical dysfunction • Cardiovascular disease • Atherosclerosis • Biliary stasis • Insulin resistance • Poor metabolism and utilization of fats • Fatty liver • Early stage hyperglycemia/Diabetes • Metabolic Syndrome • Hyperlipoproteinemia • Multiple sclerosis
	Low	• Oxidative stress • Heavy metal body burden • Liver/biliary dysfunction • Diet- malnutrition • Thyroid hyperfunction • Autoimmune processes • Adrenal hyperfunction
LDL	High	• Diet- high in refined carbohydrates • Metabolic Syndrome • Atherosclerosis • Fatty liver/Hyperlipidemia • Oxidative stress
HDL	High	• Autoimmune processes
	Low	• Hyperlipidemia • Atherosclerosis • Metabolic Syndrome • Oxidative stress • Heavy metals • Fatty liver • Hyperthyroidism • Lack of exercise/sedentary lifestyle
BUN	High	• Renal disease • Renal insufficiency • Dehydration • Hypochlorhydria • Diet- excessive protein intake • Adrenal hyperfunction • Dysbiosis • Edema • Anterior pituitary dysfunction
	Low	• Diet- low protein • Malabsorption • Pancreatic insufficiency • Liver dysfunction

263

COMPONENT	HIGH/LOW	CONDITION
Creatinine	**High**	• BPH • Urinary tract congestion • Renal disease • Renal insufficiency • Uterine hypertrophy
	Low	• Muscle atrophy
Bun/Creatinine ratio	**High**	• Renal disease
	Low	• Diet- low protein • Posterior pituitary dysfunction
Uric Acid	**High**	• Gout • Atherosclerosis/Oxidative stress • Rheumatoid arthritis • Renal insufficiency • Renal disease • Circulatory disorders • Leaky gut syndrome
	Low	• Molybdenum deficiency • Anemia- B12/folate deficiency • Copper deficiency
Potassium	**High**	• Adrenal hypofunction • Dehydration • Tissue destruction • Metabolic acidosis
	Low	• Adrenal hyperfunction • Drug diuretics • Benign essential hypertension
Sodium	**High**	• Adrenal hyperfunction • Cushing's disease • Dehydration
	Low	• Adrenal hypofunction • Addison's disease • Edema • Drug diuretics
Chloride	**High**	• Metabolic acidosis • Adrenal hyperfunction
	Low	• Hypochlorhydria • Metabolic alkalosis • Adrenal hypofunction
CO2	**High**	• Metabolic alkalosis • Adrenal hyperfunction • Hypochlorhydria • Respiratory acidosis
	Low	• Metabolic acidosis • Thiamine need • Respiratory alkalosis

COMPONENT	HIGH/LOW	CONDITION
Anion Gap	High	• Thiamine need • Metabolic acidosis
Total Protein	High	• Dehydration
	Low	• Hypochlorhydria • Digestive dysfunction and/or inflammation • Liver dysfunction • Diet- protein malnutrition/amino acid need
Albumin	High	• Dehydration
	Low	• Hypochlorhydria • Liver dysfunction • Oxidative stress • Vitamin C need
Globulin	High	• Hypochlorhydria • Liver cell damage • Oxidative stress • Heavy metal toxicity
	Low	• Digestive dysfunction and/or inflammation • Immune insufficiency
Albumin/ Globulin ratio	Low	• Liver dysfunction • Immune activation
Calcium	High	• Parathyroid hyperfunction • Thyroid hypofunction • Impaired membrane health
	Low	• Parathyroid hypofunction • Calcium need • Hypochlorhydria
Phosphorous	High	• Parathyroid hypofunction • Bone growth and/or repair • Diet- excessive phosphorous consumption • Renal insufficiency
	Low	• Parathyroid hyperfunction • Hypochlorhydria • Hyperinsulinism • Diet- high in refined carbohydrates
Magnesium	High	• Renal dysfunction • Thyroid hypofunction
	Low	• Epilepsy • Muscle spasm
Alkaline phosphatase	High	• Biliary obstruction • Liver cell damage • Bone: loss/increased turnover or bone growth and/or repair • Leaky gut syndrome • Herpes zoster • Metastatic carcinoma of the bone
	Low	• Zinc deficiency

COMPONENT	HIGH/LOW	CONDITION
SGOT/AST	High	• Dysfunction located outside of the liver and Biliary tree • Developing Congestive Heart Failure • Acute MI • Cardiovascular dysfunction: Coronary artery insufficiency • Liver cell damage • Liver dysfunction • Excess muscle breakdown or turnover • Infectious mononucleosis, EBV, CMV
	Low	• B6 deficiency • Alcoholism
SGPT/ALT	High	• Dysfunction located in the liver • Fatty liver • Liver dysfunction • Biliary tract obstruction • Excessive muscle breakdown or turnover • Cirrhosis of the liver • Liver cell damage
	Low	• B6 deficiency • Fatty liver (early development) • Liver congestion • Alcoholism
GGTP	High	• Dysfunction located outside the liver and inside the biliary tree • Biliary obstruction • Biliary stasis/insufficiency • Liver cell damage • Alcoholism • Acute/chronic Pancreatitis • Pancreatic insufficiency
	Low	• B6 deficiency • Magnesium need
LDH	High	• Liver/biliary dysfunction • Cardiovascular disease • Anemia- B12/folate deficiency, hemolytic • Non-specific tissue inflammation • Tissue destruction • Viral infection
	Low	• Reactive hypoglycemia
Total Bilirubin	High	• Biliary stasis • Oxidative stress • Thymus dysfunction • Biliary tract obstruction or calculi • Liver dysfunction • RBC hemolysis • Gilbert's syndrome
	Low	• Spleen insufficiency

Blood Chemistry and CBC Interpretation- **Patterns**

COMPONENT	HIGH/LOW	CONDITION
Direct Bilirubin	High	• Biliary tract obstruction • Biliary calculi/obstruction (usually extra hepatic)
Indirect Bilirubin	High	• RBC hemolysis • Gilbert's syndrome
Serum Iron	High	• Liver dysfunction • Hemochromatosis/hemosiderosis/iron overload • Iron conversion problem • Viral infection • Excess iron consumption
	Low	• Anemia- iron deficiency • Hypochlorhydria • Internal/microscopic bleeding
Ferritin	High	• Hemochromatosis/hemosiderosis/iron overload • Excess iron consumption • Inflammation/liver dysfunction/oxidative stress
	Low	• Anemia- iron deficiency
TIBC	High	• Anemia- iron deficiency • Internal bleeding
	Low	• Hemochromatosis/hemosiderosis/iron overload • Microscopic bleeding • Diet- protein malnutrition
% Transferrin Saturation	High	• Hemochromatosis/hemosiderosis/iron overload
	Low	• Anemia- iron deficiency
TSH	High	• Primary hypothyroidism
	Low	• Hyperthyroidism • Secondary hypothyroidism- anterior pituitary dysfunction • Tertiary hypothyroidism- hypothalamic dysfunction • Heavy metal body burden
T-3	High	• Hyperthyroidism • Iodine deficiency
	Low	• Primary hypothyroidism • Selenium deficiency
T-4	High	• Hyperthyroidism • Thyroid hormone replacement
	Low	• Primary hypothyroidism • Iodine deficiency
T-3 Uptake	High	• Hyperthyroidism • Thyroid hormone replacement
	Low	• Primary hypothyroidism • Secondary hypothyroidism- anterior pituitary dysfunction • Selenium deficiency • Iodine deficiency
ESR	High	• Non-specific tissue inflammation or destruction

Complete Blood Count

COMPONENT	HIGH/LOW	CONDITION
White Blood Cell Count	High	• Childhood diseases (Measles, Mumps, Rubella, Chicken pox etc.) • Acute bacterial infection • Acute viral infection • Stress • Diet- High in refined carbohydrates
	Low	• Chronic viral infections • Chronic bacterial infections • Leukocytic auto-digestion • Systemic Lupus Erythematosis (SLE) • Decreased production from bone marrow • Diet- raw food diet
Red Blood Cell Count	High	• Respiratory distress: Asthma or emphysema • Polycythemia (relative or absolute) • Dehydration
	Low	• Anemia- Iron deficiency • Anemia- B12/folate deficiency • Anemia- Copper deficiency • Internal bleeding • Vitamin C need
Hemoglobin	High	• Respiratory distress: Asthma or emphysema • Polycythemia (relative or primary) • Dehydration
	Low	• Anemia- iron deficiency • Anemia- B12/folate deficiency • Anemia- B6 deficiency anemia • Anemia- Copper deficiency • Internal bleeding • Digestive inflammation • Vitamin C need
Hematocrit	High	• Respiratory distress: Asthma or emphysema • Polycythemia (relative or primary) • Spleen hyperfunction • Dehydration
	Low	• Anemia • Anemia- Iron deficiency • Anemia- B12/folate deficiency • Anemia- B6 deficiency • Anemia- Copper deficiency • Internal bleeding • Digestive inflammation • Thymus hypofunction • Vitamin C need

COMPONENT	HIGH/LOW	CONDITION
MCV	High	• Anemia- B12/folate deficiency • Vitamin C need
	Low	• Anemia- Iron deficiency • Anemia- B6 deficiency • Internal bleeding
MCH	High	• Anemia- B12/folate deficiency • Hypochlorhydria
	Low	• Anemia- Iron deficiency • Anemia- B6 deficiency • Internal bleeding • Heavy metal body burden • Vitamin C need
MCHC	High	• Anemia- B12/folate deficiency • Hypochlorhydria
	Low	• Anemia- Iron deficiency • Anemia- B6 deficiency • Heavy metal body burden • Vitamin C need
RDW	High	• Anemia- Iron deficiency • Anemia- B12/folate deficiency • Pernicious anemia
Neutrophils	High	• Childhood diseases (Measles, Mumps, Rubella, Chicken pox) • Acute or chronic bacterial infection • Inflammation
	Low	• Blood diseases (aplastic anemia, pernicious anemia etc.) • Chronic viral infection
Bands	High	• Active bacterial infections
Monocytes	High	• Recovery phase of infection • Liver dysfunction • Intestinal parasites • Benign Prostatic Hypertrophy (BPH)
Lymphocytes	High	• Childhood diseases (Measles, Mumps, Rubella, Chicken pox etc.) • Acute and chronic viral infection • Infectious mononucleosis • Inflammation • Systemic toxicity
	Low	• Chronic viral or bacterial infections • Free radical activity • Active bacterial infection • Suppressed bone marrow function
Eosinophils	High	• Intestinal parasites • Food and environmental allergies/sensitivities • Asthma
	Low	• Increased adrenal steroid production

269

COMPONENT	HIGH/LOW	CONDITION
Basophils	High	• Tissue inflammation • Intestinal parasites
Platelet count	High	• Atherosclerosis
	Low	• Idiopathic thrombocytopenia • Heavy metal body burden • Free radical pathology
Reticulocytes	High	• Internal or microscopic bleeding • Anemia- hemolytic
	Low	• Iron deficiency or aplastic anemia

Section Two

The second section is the common patterns arranged by conditions. Beside each condition is a list of the patterns organized by which components of the blood chemistry screen and complete blood count are high or low for any given condition.

CONDITION	HIGH	LOW
Adrenal hyperfunction	↑ Sodium ↑ Chloride ↑ CO2 ↑ BUN	↓ Potassium ↓ Cholesterol ↓ Triglyceride
Adrenal hypofunction	↑ Potassium ↑ Cholesterol ↑ Triglycerides	↓ Sodium ↓ Chloride ↓ Blood Glucose
Anemia- B12/folate deficiency	↑ MCH ↑ MCV ↑ RDW ↑ serum iron ↑ LDH	↓ RBCs ↓ HCT ↓ HGB ↓ WBCs ↓Neutrophils ↓ Uric acid
Anemia- B6 deficiency (confirm with a serum or urinary homocysteine)	↑ or **N** HGB ↑ or **N** Serum iron increased.,	↓ MCV ↓ MCH ↓ MCHC ↓ HCT ↓ HGB ↓ or **N** SGPT/ALT ↓ <10 SGOT/AST
Anemia- Copper deficiency	Low high MCV, ↑ to **N** MCH, ↑ hair copper.	↓ HCT ↓HGB ↓ RBC ↓ Hair copper
Anemia- hemolytic	↑ LDH ↑ Reticulocytes	
Anemia- Iron deficiency	↑ TIBC ↑ Transferrin, **If hypochlorhydria is present:** ↑ Globulin 2.8	↓ Serum iron ↓ Ferritin ↓ % transferrin saturation ↓ or **N** RBCs, HGB and HCT ↓ MCV, ↓ MCH, ↓ MCHC ↓ Globulin ↓ Phosphorous

CONDITION	HIGH	LOW
Anterior pituitary/secondary thyroid hypofunction	↑ Triglycerides ↑ Cholesterol ↑ BUN	↓TSH ↓ T-3 uptake
Arthritis	↑ ESR ↑ C-reactive protein ↑ or **N** albumin ↑ Globulin ↑ Platelets	↓ or **N** albumin
Asthma	↑ HGB ↑ Eosinophils ↑ HCT, ↑ Neutrophils ↑ or **N** Total WBC	↓ lymphocytes ↓ Plasma and salivary cortisol in the chronic phase.
Atherosclerosis	↑ Triglycerides ↑ or **N** cholesterol ↑ LDL ↑ Uric acid ↑ Platelets ↑ C reactive protein	↓ HDL cholesterol
Autoimmune processes-tissue destruction	↑ HDL ↑ LDH	↓ Triglycerides ↓ or **N** Cholesterol
B6 deficiency	↑ or **N** HGB ↑ or **N** Serum iron increased.,	↓ MCV ↓ MCH ↓ MCHC ↓ HCT ↓ HGB ↓ or **N** SGPT/ALT ↓ <10 SGOT/AST
Biliary dysfunction	↑ Alkaline phosphatase ↑ GGTP ↑ SGPT/ALT ↑ LDH	↓ Triglycerides ↓ Cholesterol
Biliary obstruction/calculi	↑ Alkaline phosphatase ↑ SGPT/ALT ↑ GGTP ↑ Bilirubin ↑ Direct bilirubin	
Biliary stasis/insufficiency	↑ Cholesterol ↑ GGTP ↑ Bilirubin	
BPH	↑ Creatinine ↑ PSA (may be normal) ↑ Monocytes	
Cardiovascular disease	↑ Triglycerides ↑ Cholesterol ↑ LDL ↑ LDH ↑ SGOT/AST	↓ HDL

CONDITION	HIGH	LOW
Childhood diseases	↑ WBC ↑ Neutrophil (early) ↑ Lymphocytes (later)	↓ Neutrophils (later) ↓ Lymphocytes (early)
Copper deficiency	Low high MCV, ↑ to **N** MCH,	↓ HCT ↓HGB ↓ RBC ↓ Uric acid
Deficient Red Blood Cell production	↑ Serum iron	↓ RBC ↓ HCT
Dehydration	↑ RBC count ↑ HGB ↑ HCT ↑ Total protein (Chronic) ↑ Albumin (Chronic) ↑ Sodium ↑ Potassium ↑ BUN (Chronic)	
Diabetes/hyperglycemia	↑ Blood Glucose ↑ Hemoglobin A1C ↑ Cholesterol ↑ Triglycerides	
Diet- fat deficient		↓ Cholesterol ↓ Triglycerides
Diet- high in refined carbohydrates	↑ LDL Cholesterol	↓ Phosphorous Total WBC count
Diet- low protein		↓ BUN ↓ Total protein ↓ BUN-Creatinine ratio
Digestive dysfunction/inflammation	↑ or **N** MCV ↑ or **N** MCH ↑ total globulin ↑ BUN ↑ Basophils **With Ulceration or erosion:** ↑ Alk Phos intestinal isoenzyme	↓ Total protein ↓ Albumin ↓ Phosphorous ↓ HCT ↓ HGB
Edema	↑ BUN	↓ Sodium
Emphysema	↑ HCT ↑ RBCs ↑ or **N** CO_2 ↑ or **N** RBC	↓↓ Alpha I globulin ↓ or **N** serum chloride
Excess consumption of iron	↑ Serum iron ↑ Ferritin	
Fatty liver	↑ Blood Glucose ↑ Triglycerides ↑ Cholesterol ↑ LDL Cholesterol	↓ HDL Cholesterol ↓ SGPT/ALT
Gilbert's syndrome	↑ Bilirubin ↑ Indirect bilirubin	

272

CONDITION	HIGH	LOW
Gout	↑ Uric acid ↑ Cholesterol ↑ BUN ↑ or **N** Creatinine	↓ Phosphorous
Heavy metal burden (run a hair/urine analysis if this pattern comes up to rule this out)	↑ Uric acid ↑ Total bilirubin ↑ BUN Cadmium toxicity: ↑ Calcium	↓ MCHC and MCH ↓ HCT and HGB ↓ RBC ↓ 5th Isoenzyme of LDH Cadmium toxicity: ↓ Phosphorous
Heavy metals/chemical toxicity	↓ Cholesterol ↓ HDL Cholesterol ↑ Total globulin ↓ TSH	↓ MCH ↓ MCHC ↓ Platelets
Hemochromatosis	↑ Serum iron ↑ Ferritin ↑ % Transferrin saturation	↓ TIBC
Hyperinsulinemia	↓ Blood Glucose ↑ Triglycerides ↑ Cholesterol	↓ HDL Cholesterol ↓ Phosphorous
Hyperlipidemia	↑ Triglycerides ↑ Cholesterol ↑ LDL Cholesterol	↓ HDL Cholesterol
Hyperlipoproteinemia	↑ Triglycerides ↑ Cholesterol	
Hypochlorhydria	↑ BUN ↑ MCV ↑ MCH ↑ MCHC ↑ CO_2 ↑ Total globulin	↓ Chloride ↓ Anion gap ↓ or **N** Calcium ↓ Phosphorous ↓ or **N** Serum iron ↓ Total globulin (2°) ↓ Alkaline phosphatase ↓ or **N** Total protein ↓ or **N** Albumin
Hypoglycemia- liver glycogen storage problem	↑ SGPT/ALT	↓ Blood Glucose ↓ Hemoglobin A1C ↓ LDH
Hypoglycemia- reactive		↓ Blood Glucose ↓ Hemoglobin A1C ↓ LDH
Increased Red blood cell destruction	↑ Bilirubin (> 1.2) ↑ Indirect bilirubin	↓ RBC
Infection: active	↑ WBCs ↑ Neutrophils ↑ Bands ↑ ESR	↓ Lymphocytes

CONDITION	HIGH	LOW
Infection: Acute bacterial	↑ WBCs ↑ Neutrophils ↑ Monocytes (recovery phase) ↑ Bands ↑ ESR	↓ or **N** Lymphocytes
Infection: Acute viral	↑ WBCs ↑ Lymphocytes ↑ Monocytes (recovery phase) ↑ Bands ↑ ESR ↑ LDH	↓ or **N** Neutrophils
Infection: Chronic viral	↑ Serum iron	↓ WBCs ↓ Lymphocytes
Inflammation- non-specific	↑ LDH ↑ ESR ↑ Ferritin ↑ Basophils	
Insulin Resistance	↑ Blood Glucose ↑ Hemoglobin A1C ↑ Triglycerides ↑ Cholesterol	
Internal bleeding	↑ Reticulocyte count ↑ TIBC ↑ Transferrin.	↓ or **N** serum iron ↓ or **N** serum ferritin ↓ HGB ↓ or **N** HCT ↓ MCV ↓ MCH
Internal microscopic bleeding	↑ Reticulocyte count	↓ TIBC ↓ Transferrin
Intestinal parasites	↑ Eosinophils ↑ or **N** Basophils ↑ or **N** Monocytes ↑ IgE Stool positive for parasites or ova	↓ or **N** serum iron ↓ or **N** HGB ↓ or **N** HCT
Iodine deficiency	↑ T-3	↓ T-3 uptake ↓ T-4
Iron deficiency	↑ TIBC ↑ Transferrin, If hypochlorhydria is present: ↑ Globulin 2.8	↓ Serum iron ↓ Ferritin ↓ % transferrin saturation ↓ or **N** RBCs, HGB and HCT ↓ MCV, ↓ MCH, ↓ MCHC ↓ Globulin ↓ Phosphorous
Leaky gut syndrome	↑ Uric acid ↑ Alkaline phosphatase	

CONDITION	HIGH	LOW
Liver cell damage	↑ Total globulin ↑ Alkaline phosphatase ↑ SGOT/AST ↑ SGPT/ALT ↑ GGTP	
Liver dysfunction	↑ SGPT/ALT ↑ LDH ↑ SGOT/AST ↑ Bilirubin ↑ Direct bilirubin ↑ Serum iron ↑ Ferritin ↑ Monocytes	↓ BUN ↓ Total protein ↓ Albumin ↓ Albumin/globulin ratio ↓ Triglycerides ↓ Cholesterol
Malabsorption		↓ BUN ↓ GGTP
Metabolic acidosis	↑ Chloride ↑ Anion gap ↑ Potassium	↓ CO_2
Metabolic alkalosis	↑ CO_2	↓ Chloride ↓ Calcium ↓ Potassium
Microscopic bleeding	↑ Reticulocytes	↓ TIBC
Mononucleosis	↑ SGOT/AST ↑ Alkaline phosphatase ↑ LDH ↑ WBCs (2nd week) ↑ GGTP ↑ Lymphocytes	↓ WBCs (1st week)
Muscle- atrophy or breakdown	↑ SGOT/AST ↑ SGPT/ALT	↓ Creatinine

Neoplasms
(A pattern potentially seen with developing neoplasms)
	↑ or ↓ total WBC in conjunction with:
	    ↓ lymphocyte (<20)
	    ↓ serum albumin (4.0)
	If this pattern does not change after 30 days on a supplemental program/prescribed drugs, Further evaluation to rule out neoplasm should be considered.	

Oxidative stress/Free radical activity	↑ LDL Cholesterol ↑ Uric acid ↑ Total globulin ↑ Bilirubin ↑ Ferritin ↑ Platelets	↓ Lymphocytes ↓ Cholesterol (below historical average) ↓ HDL Cholesterol ↓ Albumin
Pancreatic insufficiency	↑ GGTP	↓ Total WBC count ↓ BUN

275

CONDITION	HIGH	LOW
Parasites- intestinal	↑ Monocytes ↑ Basophils ↑ Eosinophils	
Parathyroid hyperfunction	↑ Calcium	↓ Phosphorous
Parathyroid hypofunction	↑ Phosphorous	↓ Calcium
Polycythemia	↑ RBCs ↑ HCT ↑ HGB ↑ Total bilirubin ↑ Uric acid ↑ WBC ↑ Basophils ↑ Alk phos	↓ or **N** MCV ↓ or **N** MCH ↓ or **N** serum iron
Poor fat metabolism	↑ Triglycerides ↑ Cholesterol	
Posterior pituitary dysfunction		↓ BUN ↓ BUN-Creatinine ratio
Pregnancy	↑ Total cholesterol ↑ MCV and MCH ↑ Neutrophils ↑ T-4 ↑ Total WBCs (late)	↓ calcium in late pregnancy ↓ albumin ↓ HGB and HCT ↓ T-3 uptake ↓ Lymphocytes (late)) ↓ Total protein
Renal disease	↑ Uric acid ↑ Phosphorous ↑ LDH ↑ SGOT/AST ↑ BUN ↑ Creatinine ↑ BUN-Creatinine ratio ↑ Magnesium	
Renal insufficiency	↑ BUN ↑ or **N** Creatinine ↑ or **N** Uric acid ↑ Phosphorous	
Respiratory distress	↑ RBCs ↑ HGB ↑ HCT ↑ Eosinophils	
Rheumatoid arthritis	↑ Uric acid ↑ ESR	↓ or **N** albumin ↓ or **N** albumin
Selenium deficiency		↓ T-3 ↓ T-3 uptake
Suppressed bone marrow production		↓ in all white blood cells ↓ RBCs ↓ HCT ↓ HGB

CONDITION	HIGH	LOW
Metabolic Syndrome	↑ Blood Glucose ↑ Triglycerides ↑ Cholesterol ↑ LDL	↓ HDL Cholesterol
Systemic Lupus Erythematosus (SLE)	↑ ANA ↑ ESR ↑ SGPT/ALT ↑ C-reactive protein ↑ Alpha 1 globulin ↑ Gamma globulin ↑ IgA, IgG, IgM and IgD ↑ IgG in initial stages ↑ IgA as disease progresses	↓ Total WBC count ↓ to **N** lymphocytes ↓ Serum albumin ↓ C-complement ↓ IgG as disease progresses ↓ IgA in initial stages ↓ HCT, RBCs and HGB
Systemic toxicity	↑ Lymphocytes	
Thiamine deficiency	↑ Blood Glucose ↑ Anion Gap	↓ CO2
Thymus dysfunction	↑ Bilirubin ↑ HGB ↑ HCT ↑ RBCs	↓ Hematocrit
Thyroid hormone replacement	↑ T-4 ↑ T-3 uptake	
Thyroid hyperfunction	↑ T-3 ↑ T-4 ↑ T-3 uptake	↓ Triglycerides ↓ Cholesterol ↓ HDL Cholesterol ↓ TSH
Thyroid hypofunction- primary	↑ TSH ↑ Triglycerides ↑ Cholesterol ↑ Calcium ↑ Magnesium	↓ T-3 ↓ T-4 ↓ T-3 uptake
Thyroid hypofunction- secondary due to anterior pituitary dysfunction	↑ Triglycerides ↑ Cholesterol ↑ BUN	↓ TSH ↓ T-3 uptake
Tissue destruction	↑ Potassium ↑ LDH ↑ ESR	
Tissue inflammation/ destruction (GI, tendon/bursa, phlebitis, sinusitis, musculoskeletal)	↑ ESR ↑ Potassium ↑ Basophils ↑ ALP increased with liver, bone or gastric inflammation.	
Urinary tract congestion	↑ Creatinine ↑ Monocytes	

CONDITION	HIGH	LOW
Vitamin B12/folate deficiency	↑ MCH ↑ MCV ↑ RDW ↑ serum iron ↑ LDH	↓ RBCs ↓ HCT ↓ HGB ↓ WBCs ↓ Neutrophils ↓ Uric acid
Vitamin B6 deficiency		↓ SGOT/AST ↓ SGPT/ALT ↓ GGTP
Vitamin C need	↑ MCV ↑ Alk Phos ↑ Fibrinogen	↓ Albumin ↓ MCH ↓ MCHC ↓ HGB ↓ HCT ↓ RBCs ↓ Serum iron
Zinc deficiency		↓ Alkaline phosphatase

<u>Bibliography of Works Consulted</u>

Batmanghelidj, F, M.D., *Your Body's Many Cries for Water.*

Berkow, Robert, M.D., editor in chief. *The Merck Manual*, 16th ed. Rahway, N.J.

Braunwald, Eugene, et al. *Harrison's Principles of Internal Medicine*. 13th ed. New York: McGraw-Hill Book Co.: 1999.

Coca, Arthur M.D., *The Pulse Test*. St. Martins Press, New York. 1994.

Collins, John, N.D. "Gastroenterology" class notes and handouts. Portland, OR: National College of Naturopathic Medicine; 1998.

DeGowin, Richard L., M.D.; *Bedside Diagnostic Examination*. Sixth ed. New York: McGraw Hill. 1997.

Erasmus, Udo. *Fats that Heal, Fats that Kill.* Alive Books Press, Vancouver B.C., 1986.

Fischbach, Frances. *A Manual of Laboratory & Diagnostic Tests* (Fifth edition). New York: Lippincott, 1996.

Gottschall, Elaine, B.A., M.Sc. *Breaking the Vicious Cycle.*

Harrower, Henry, M.D. *Practical Endocrinology*. Glendale, CA: Pioneer Printing Company, Inc., 1982.

Jamieson, T.K., D.O., Duffy, Daniel, D.C. *Balancing Body Chemistry With Nutrition: A Manual for Metabolic/Nutritional Evaluation of the SMA/25*, Cannonsburg, MI, 1996.

Marz, R; *Medical Nutrition from Marz*. 2nd ed. Portland, OR; 1998.

Owens, Charles. *An Endocrine Interpretation of Chapman's Reflexes*. American Academy of Osteopathy, Newark, Ohio, 1937. Reprinted 1994.

Pizzorno, Joseph E, ND; Murray, Michal, ND. *Textbook of Natural Medicine*. Seattle: John Bastyr College Publications; 1985.

Pottenger, Francis M., M.D.; *Pottenger's Cats – A Study in Nutrition*. 2nd edition. 1995.

Price, Weston. *Nutrition and Physical Degeneration*. Price-Pottenger Nutrition Foundation, Inc. 1997.

Ravel, Richard. *Clinical Laboratory Medicine*. (Sixth edition). Boston, Mosby, 1995.

Tortora, Gerald J: Anagoustakos, N.P. *Principles of Anatomy and Physiology, 7th* ed. New York: Harper and Row Publishers; 1997.

Walther, David S.; *Applied Kinesiology – Synopsis*. Systems DC press. 1988.

Yanick Jr., Paul, PhD; Jaffe, Russell, M.D., PhD., editors. *Clinical Chemistry and Nutrition Guidebook: A Physician's Desk Reference*, Volume One. T & H Publishing; 1988.

CHEMSCREEN and CBC RESULTS TRACKING FORM STANDARD U.S. UNITS

NAME: DATE:

TEST	REF. RANGE	RESULT	OPTIMAL	↓/↑	NOTES
Glucose	65 – 115		80 – 100		
HgB A1C	<7%		4.1 – 5.7%		
BUN	5 – 25		10 – 16		
Creatinine	0.6 – 1.5		0.8 – 1.1		
Sodium	135 – 147		135 – 142		
Potassium	3.5 – 5.3		4.0 – 4.5		
Chloride	96 – 109		100 – 106		
CO_2	22 – 32		25 – 30		
Anion Gap	6 – 16		7 – 12		
Uric Acid	2.2 – 7.7		3.5 – 5.9 male 3.0 –5.5 female		
Total Protein	6.0 – 8.5		6.9 – 7.4		
Albumin	3.5 – 5.5		4.0 – 5.0		
Calcium	8.5 – 10.8		9.2 – 10.0		
Phosphorous	2.5 – 4.5		3.0 – 4.0		
Alk Phos	25 – 140		70 – 100		
SGOT(AST)	0 – 40		10 – 30		
SGPT(ALT)	0 – 45		10 – 30		
LDH	1 – 240		140 – 200		
total Bilirubin direct indirect	0.1 – 1.2 0 – 0.2 0.1 – 1.0		0.1 – 1.2 (>2.6) 0 – 0.2 (>0.8) 0.1 – 1.0 (>1.8)		
GGTP	1 – 70		10 – 30		
Globulin	2.0 – 3.9		2.4 – 2.8		
A/G ratio	1.0 – 2.4		1.4 – 2.1		
BUN/Creat.	7 – 18		10 – 16		
Total iron	30 – 170		50 – 100		
Cholesterol	130 – 200		150 – 220		
Triglycerides	30 – 150		70 – 110		
LDL	60 – 130		<120		
HDL	40 – 90		>55		
Chol/HDL	Ratio		<4		
Ferritin	33 - 236 10 - 122		33 – 236 male 10 – 122 female		
TIBC	250 – 350		250 – 350		
TSH	0.35 – 5.50		2.0 – 4.4		
T-3 uptake	22 – 39		27 – 37		
T-3	80 – 230		100 – 230		
T-4 thyroxine	4.8 – 13.2		6 – 12		
FTI/ T-7	1.2 – 4.9		6.0 – 11.0		
COMPLETE BLOOD COUNT					
WBC	3.7 – 10.5		5.0 – 7.5		
RBC	4.1 – 5.6 3.8 – 5.1		4.2 – 4.9 male 3.9 – 4.5 fem		
Reticulocyte	0.5 – 1		0.5 – 1		
Hemoglobin	12.5 – 17.0 11.5 – 15.0		14 – 15 male 13.5 – 14.5 fem		
Hematocrit	36 – 50% 34 – 44		40 – 48 male 37 – 4 4 female		
MCV	80 – 98		82 – 89.9		
MCH	27 – 34		28 – 31.9		
MCHC	32 – 36		32 – 35		
Platelets	155 – 385		150 – 385 x 1000		
RDW	11.7 – 15.0		<13		
Neutrophils	40 – 74%		40 – 60%		
Lymphs	14 – 46%		24 – 44%		
Monocytes	4 – 13%		0 – 7%		
Eosinophils	0 – 7%		0 – 3%		
Basophils	0 – 3%		0 – 1%		

CONVERSION CHART FOR CONVERTING STANDARD US UNITS INTO STANDARD INTERNATIONAL UNITS

TEST	US UNITS	CONVERSION FACTOR → Multiply ← Divide	S.I. UNITS
Glucose	mg/dL	0.05551	mmol/L
HgB A1C	%	0.01	
BUN	mg/dL	0.357	mmol/L
Creatinine	mg/dL	88.4	μmol/dL
Sodium	mEq/L	1	mmol/L
Potassium	mEq/L	1	mmol/L
Chloride	mEq/L	1	mmol/L
CO_2	mEq/L	1	mmol/L
Anion Gap	mEq/L	1	mmol/L
Uric Acid	mg/dL	59.48	μmol/dL
Total Protein	g/dL	10	g/L
Albumin	g/dL	10	g/L
Calcium	mg/dL	0.250	mmol/L
Phosphorous	mg/dL	0.3229	mmol/L
Alk Phos	U/L	1	U/L
SGOT(AST)	U/L	1	U/L
SGPT(ALT)	U/L	1	U/L
LDH	U/L	1	U/L
Bilirubin values	mg/dL	17.1	μmol/dL
GGTP	U/L	1	U/L
Globulin	g/dL	10	g/L
A/G ratio	Ratio	1	Ratio
BUN/Creat.	Ratio	1	Ratio
Total iron	mg/dL	0.1791	μmol/dL
Cholesterol	mg/dL	0.02586	mmol/L
Triglycerides	mg/dL	0.01129	mmol/L
LDL	mg/dL	0.02586	mmol/L
HDL	mg/dL	0.02586	mmol/L
Chol/HDL	Ratio	1	Ratio
Ferritin	ng/mL	1	μg/L
TIBC	μg/dL	0.1791	μmol/dL
TSH	μIU/mL	1	mIU/L
T-3 uptake	%	0.01	%
T-3	ng/dL	0.01536	nmol/L
T-4 thyroxine	μg/dL	12.87	nmol/L
FTI/ T-7		1	
WBC	x 10^3/mm^3	1	10^9/L
RBC	x 10^6/mm^3	1	10^{12}/L
Hemoglobin	g/dL	10	g/L
Hematocrit	%	0.01	1
MCV	Microns^3	1	fL
MCH	pg	1	pg
MCHC	g/dL	1	1
Platelets	x 10^3/mm^3	1	10^9/L
RDW	Calculated	1	Calculated
Neutrophils	%	1	%
Lymphs	%	1	%
Monocytes	%	1	%
Eosinophils	%	1	%
Basophils	%	1	%

CHEMSCREEN and CBC RESULTS TRACKING FORM STANDARD INTERNATIONAL UNITS

NAME: DATE:

TEST	REF. RANGE	RESULT	OPTIMAL	↓/↑
Glucose	3.61 – 6.38		4.44 – 5.55	
HgB A1C	<0.07		0.041 – 0.057	
BUN	1.79 – 8.93		3.57 – 5.71	
Creatinine	53.0 – 132.6		70.7 – 97.2	
Sodium	135 – 147		135 – 142	
Potassium	3.5 – 5.3		4.0 – 4.5	
Chloride	96 – 109		100 – 106	
CO_2	22 – 32		25 – 30	
Anion Gap	6 – 16		7 – 12	
Uric Acid	131 – 458		208 – 351 male 178 – 327 female	
Total Protein	60 – 85		69 – 74	
Albumin	35 – 55		40 – 50	
Calcium	2.13 – 2.70		2.30 – 2.50	
Phosphorous	0.81 – 1.45		0.97 – 1.29	
Alk Phos	25 – 140		70 – 100	
SGOT(AST)	0 – 40		10 – 30	
SGPT(ALT)	0 – 45		10 – 30	
LDH	1 – 240		140 – 200	
total Bilirubin direct indirect	1.7 – 20.5 0 – 3.4 1.7 – 17.1		1.7 – 20.5 (>44.5) 0 – 3.4 (>13.7) 1.7 – 17.1 (>30.8)	
GGTP	1 – 70		10 – 30	
Globulin	20 – 39		24 – 28	
A/G ratio	1.1 – 2.5		1.5 – 2.0	
BUN/Creat.	7 – 14		13 – 17	
Total iron	5.37 – 30.45		8.96 – 17.91	
Cholesterol	3.36 – 5.20		3.9 – 5.69	
Triglycerides	0.34 – 1.7		0.79 – 1.24	
LDL	1.55 – 3.36		<3.1	
HDL	1.03 – 2.32		>1.42	
Chol/HDL	Ratio		<4	
Ferritin	33 - 236 10 - 122		33 – 236 male 10 – 122 female	
TIBC	44.8 – 62.7		44.8 – 62.7	
TSH	0.35 – 5.50		2.0 – 4.4	
T-3 uptake	22 – 39		27 – 37	
T-3	1.23 – 3.53		1.54 – 3.53	
T-4 thyroxine	61.8 – 169.9		77.2 – 154.4	
FTI/ T-7	1.2 – 4.9		6.0 – 11.0	
COMPLETE BLOOD COUNT				
WBC	3.7 – 10.5		5.0 – 7.5	
RBC	4.1 – 5.6 3.8 – 5.1		4.2 – 4.9 male 3.9 – 4.5 fem	
Reticulocyte	0.5 – 1		0.5 – 1	
Hemoglobin	125 – 170 115 – 150		140 – 150 male 135 – 145 fem	
Hematocrit	0.36 – 0.50 0.34 – 0.44		0.40 – 0.48 male 0.37 – 0.44 fem	
MCV	80 – 98		82 – 89.9	
MCH	27 – 34		28 – 31.9	
MCHC	32 – 36		32 – 35	
Platelets	155 – 385		150 – 385 x 1000	
RDW	11.7 – 15.0		<13	
Neutrophils	40 – 74%		40 – 60%	
Lymphs	14 – 46%		24 – 44%	
Monocytes	4 – 13%		0 – 7%	
Eosinophils	0 – 7%		0 – 3%	
Basophils	0 – 3%		0 – 1%	

NOTES

INDEX

C

D

286

287

U

V

W

X

Z

Books and other Resources from Bear Mountain Publishing

Blood Chemistry and CBC Analysis- Clinical Laboratory Testing from a Functional Perspective- Dicken Weatherby, N.D. and Scott Ferguson, N.D.

Quick Reference Guide to Blood Chemistry Analysis- Dicken Weatherby, N.D. and Scott Ferguson, N.D.

In-Office Laboratory Testing- Functional Terrain Analysis- Dicken Weatherby, N.D. and Scott Ferguson, N.D.

Urine Dipstick Analysis and Functional Urinalysis Quick Reference Guide- Dicken Weatherby, N.D. and Scott Ferguson, N.D.

Signs and Symptoms Analysis from a Functional Perspective- Dicken Weatherby, N.D.

Complete Physical Exam Reference and Charting System- Dicken Weatherby, N.D. and Scott Ferguson, N.D.

Complete Practitioner's Guide To Take-Home Testing- Dicken Weatherby, N.D. and Scott Ferguson, N.D.

Online Functional Blood Chemistry Analysis Training at www.BloodChemistryTraining.com

----

For more information about other titles from Bear Mountain Publishing visit us at:
http://www.BloodChemistryAnalysis.com

or e-mail us at info@BloodChemistryAnalysis.com

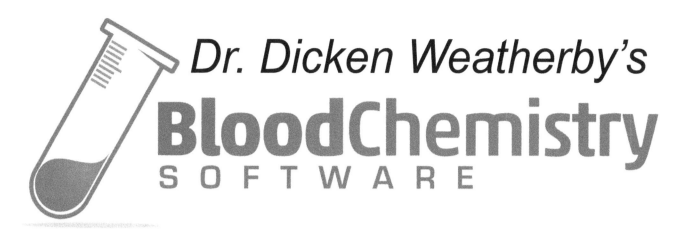

Dr. Dicken Weatherby's
BloodChemistry
SOFTWARE

"The ONLY Blood Chemistry Analysis Software Program Based EXCLUSIVELY on Dr. Weatherby's Pioneering Work Functional Blood Chemistry Analysis"

Enter & Analyze UNLIMITED Tests!

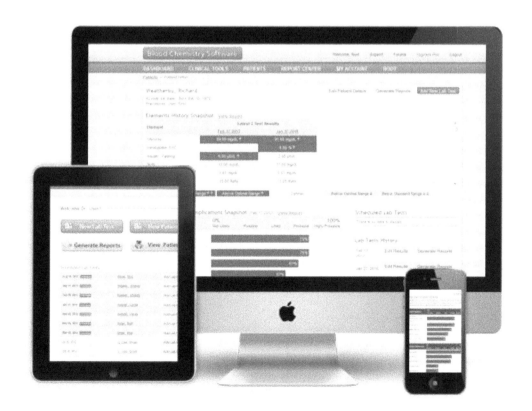

http://BloodChemSoftware.com

Blood Chemistry University™

Presented by Dr. Dicken Weatherby

Blood Chemistry University Provides You With Everything You'll Need to Be Successful........

12 "Look Over Dicken's Shoulder" Online Video Training Sessions

Lifetime Access to "Blood Chemistry University"

Audio MP3 and PDF Downloads From All Sessions!

8 Hours of Bonus Training From FM Experts

90-Days of Unlimited Software Use

4 Things You Will Know After You Join Blood Chemistry University:

☑ An understanding of the implications for blood tests that are outside the normal value and implications of blood tests that fall outside of an optimal range.

☑ A knowledge of what tests to order....You will learn what tests deserve to be on your standard panel, and what tests don't.

☑ How to turn your regular blood chemistry and CBC/Hematology test into an incredible prognostic marker for dysfunction.

☑ How to put it all together....You will have an understanding of the patterns that exist between tests and the likely dysfunctions associated with the patterns.

Dr. Weatherby's "Functional Blood Chemistry Analysis System"....What Every Health Care Practitioner Ought to Be Using In *THEIR* Functional Medicine Practices!!!"

➡ Do you want exciting new diagnostic skills to get your patients and your practice to the next level of success?

➡ Do you like rapid results and excellent clinical outcomes?

➡ Are you are looking for new tools and techniques to dramatically improve your clinical outcomes?

➡ Do you want more referrals?

➡ Do you want to take on those hard to treat cases no one else can work with?

How would you like to learn everything you need to know about the functional analysis of your patients' blood tests which will:

✔ Put you on the cutting edge of preventative diagnosis.

✔ Help you get more from the tests you are already performing.

✔ Hone your blood chemistry analysis skills.

✔ Show you how these tests can be used as a prognostic marker for dysfunction.

✔ Cut the amount of time you spend analyzing your patient's' blood tests.

http://BloodChemistryTraining.com

Lightning Source UK Ltd.
Milton Keynes UK
UKHW030630211120
373795UK00002B/32